APPROACHES TO THE TREATMENT OF APHASIA

Clinical Competence Series

Series Editor
Robert T. Wertz, Ph.D.

Approaches to the Treatment of Aphasia
Nancy Helm-Estabrooks, Sc.D., and Audrey L. Holland, Ph.D.

Manual of Articulation and Phonological Disorders
Ken M. Bleile, Ph.D.

Right Hemisphere Communication Disorders: Theory
and Management
Connie A. Tompkins, Ph.D., CCC-SLP

Manual of Voice Treatment: Pediatrics Through Geriatrics
Moya Andrews, Ed.D.

Videoendoscopy: From Velopharynx to Larynx
Michael P. Karnell, Ph.D.

Prosody Management of Communication Disorders
Patricia M. Hargrove, Ph.D., and Nancy S. McGarr, Ph.D.

Clinical Manual of Laryngectomy and Head and Neck
Cancer Rehabilitation
Janina K. Casper, Ph.D., and Raymond H. Colton, Ph.D.

Sourcebook for Medical Speech Pathology
Lee Ann C. Golper, Ph.D., CCC-SLP

APPROACHES TO THE TREATMENT OF APHASIA

Edited by

Nancy Helm-Estabrooks, Sc.D.

National Center for Neurogenic Communication Disorders
University of Arizona
Tucson

and

Department of Neurology
Boston University School of Medicine
Boston, Massachusetts

and

Audrey L. Holland, Ph.D.

Department of Speech and Hearing Sciences
University of Arizona
Tucson

SINGULAR PUBLISHING GROUP, INC.
SAN DIEGO • LONDON

COPYRIGHT © 1998
Singular Publishing Group is a division of Thomson Learning. The Thomson Learning logo is a registered trademark used herein under license.

Printed in the United States of America
3 4 5 6 7 8 9 10 XXX 05 04 03 02 01

For more information, contact Singular Publishing Group, 401 West "A" Street, Suite 325, San Diego, CA 92101-7904; or find us on the World Wide Web at http://www.singpub.com

Library of Congress Cataloging-in-Publication Data:
ISBN: 1-565-93841-0

CONTENTS

FOREWORD

com•pe•tence (kom'pə təns)   n.   The state or quality
of being properly or well qualified; capable.

Clinicians crave competence. They pursue it through education and experience,
through emulation and innovation. Some are more successful than others in attaining what they seek. This book, *Approaches to the Treatment of Aphasia,* edited by
Nancy Helm-Estabrooks and Audrey L. Holland, is designed to assist us in what
we do for adults whose language has been shattered by a neurological accident. It
is a departure from previous Singular Clinical Competence Series editions where
an author or authors have demonstrated how they manage a disorder or employ
clinical tools in patient management. Here, we have eight clinicians who have spent
considerable time knee-to-knee with aphasic people telling us how they managed
one of the hundreds of patients who have crossed their clinical thresholds. The
presentations demonstrate that the variety of treatments for aphasia is limited only
by the number of clinicians treating it. Most of all, we are reminded that there is
seldom only one way to do something well. Somewhere in each case presentation,
readers will find bits of themselves and the treatments they have administered.
Elsewhere, readers will find methods that are foreign or, to them, questionable.
That is good. If we all did the same thing for all aphasic people, treatment would
be a very dull way of spending the day. And, if we all thought alike, none of us
would be thinking. Your attention to what the authors provide indicates your competence and your effort to improve it, because competent clinicians seek competence as much for what it demands as for what it promises.

Robert T. Wertz, Ph.D.
Series Editor

PREFACE

This book is a collection of reports about how clinicians go about the clinical management of specific individuals with aphasia. The volume presents readers with an opportunity to eavesdrop on some highly experienced clinicians as they grapple with the very real problems of helping their particular patients. The eight cases presented here were first described to the other contributors to this book at a small 4-day meeting in Cody, WY in October, 1996. We discussed each case thoroughly at this "Cody Conference." As a result, each author's individual thinking has benefited from the feedback of the other participants. Carol Frattali played a somewhat different role. She was responsible for trying to keep us realistic about service delivery near the end of the 20th century. Each of the eight clinical chapters has benefited from her feedback, and she has provided commentary on our individual cases where appropriate in her chapter.

We have long shared the dream of having a truly clinical meeting, where aphasia clinicians who have a variety of approaches to the treatment of aphasia could get together with the aim of exploring clinical ideas in a leisurely manner, teaching each other, learning from each other, valuing each other's clinical insights. At Cody, we worked very hard for 4 days, but we had fun too and influenced each other's clinical thinking in many ways. Probably we all are still munching on some of the thoughts shared in Cody, and our subsequent clinical behavior has been influenced by the Cody experience. We hope that this book will stimulate your thought processes as well, and that your clinical skills will be enhanced as a result of reading it.

ACKNOWLEDGMENTS

We thank Singular Publishing Group for making the Cody Conference possible. Sadanand Singh and Marie Linvill were enthusiastic and positive supporters of our dream. We are honored by their trust and willingness to provide the financial backing for this first of what we hope will be a prototype of many such clinical conferences to come.

We also think Margaret Forbes for her help in the process of editing this book. She contributed greatly to its readability and we are deeply grateful.

CONTRIBUTORS

Pelagie Beeson, Ph.D.
Department of Speech and Hearing Sciences
University of Arizona
Tucson, Arizona

Rita Sloan Berndt, Ph.D.
Department of Neurology
University of Maryland School of Medicine
Baltimore, Maryland

Nancy Helm-Estabrooks, Sc.D.
National Center for Neurogenic Communication Disorders
University of Arizona
Tucson, Arizona
Department of Neurology
Boston University School of Medicine
Boston, Massachusetts

Carol Frattali, Ph.D.
Department of Rehabilitation Medicine
National Institutes of Health
Bethesda, Maryland

Margaret L. Greenwald, Ph.D.
Department of Psychiatry and Behavioral Neurosciences
Wayne State University
Detroit, Michigan

Audrey Holland, Ph.D.
Department of Speech and Hearing Sciences
University of Arizona
Tucson, Arizona

Jon Lyon, Ph.D.
Living with Aphasia, Inc.
Mazomanie, Wisconsin

Lynn M. Maher, Ph.D.
Department of Educational Psychology and Special Education
Georgia State University
Atlanta, Georgia

Charlotte C. Mitchum, M.S.
Department of Neurology
University of Maryland School of Medicine
Baltimore, Maryland

Cynthia Ochipa, Ph.D.
Speech-Language Pathology Service
James A. Haley Hospital
Tampa, Florida

Leslie Gonzalez Rothi, Ph.D.
Audiology and Speech Pathology Services
V.A. Medical Center
Gainesville, Florida

Cynthia Thompson, Ph.D.
Department of Communication Sciences and Disorders and Neurology Center
for Cognitive Neurology and Alzheimer's Disease
Northwestern University
Evanston, Illinois

Robert T. Wertz, Ph.D.
Audiology and Speech Pathology Services
V.A. Medical Center
Nashville, Tennessee

CHAPTER

1

The Power of One: Every Aphasia Treatment Case Is a Case Study

NANCY HELM-ESTABROOKS, Sc.D.
AUDREY L. HOLLAND, Ph.D.

I. HISTORICAL PERSPECTIVE ON CASE STUDIES

The field of clinical aphasiology was built on a foundation of case studies beginning with Paul Broca's 1865 description of the man who came to be called "Tan-Tan" in keeping with his stereotypic utterance. Published cases have contributed immeasurably to our understanding of the amazing and yet devastating phenomenon of aphasia. In like fashion, much of what we know about treatment of aphasia comes from our attempts to treat individual patients. This book is a continuation of a long tradition of clinicians sharing information about their methods for rehabilitating aphasia; a tradition that probably began in 1880. In that year, the preeminent American neurologist

Charles Mills described to a group of physicians the treatment of an aphasic patient referred to him by the English neurologist Donald Broadbent. Two years before being seen by Dr. Mills, this patient had an "attack" that left him "totally" aphasic and agraphic. His reading aloud was notable for marked paraphasia of the "jargon or gibberish type." His status on seeing Mills is uncertain, but with instruction he began to try to improve his speech and writing. He remained under Mills' care for several years and showed slow, but continuous, improvement until he was able to communicate without difficulty in both speech and writing. Mills (1880) concluded that in aphasia "much of (the recovery) is the result of methodical re-education" (p. 27). To account for this recovery he theorized that: (1) If destruction of speech centers is incomplete, part of a certain convolution may learn to do the work of the whole. (2) If centers on one side are destroyed, corresponding regions in the other hemisphere may take on the function. (3) If channels of communication are cut or blocked, new pathways may be formed.

Subsequently, Mills (1904) published a paper in the *Journal of the American Medical Association* based on an oral presentation to other physicians in which he described specific remediation techniques for different forms of aphasia. Included in that paper was the case of a 45-year-old man (also a physician) whom Mills saw in July, 1902, 18 months after the onset of right hemiplegia with complete aphasia. When seen by Mills, the man's speech consisted chiefly of nouns and verbs, with occasional use of pronouns and no use of auxiliary verbs (we would describe this patient as having agrammatic aphasia). At once a systematic and progressive course of training was instituted with the assistance of the neurologist Dr. T. H. Weisenburg and the patient's secretary. In the early stages, the training program made great use of repetition guided by Wyllie's physiologic alphabet (1894), which guided the formation of speech sounds. Next, they used a phonetic reader in which the sounds of letters and combinations were taught by special associations with objects and then used in sentences advancing from simple to more complex forms. This was followed by work with a dictionary, a language primer, and a grammar book. Later, the patient came to be under the care of another physician who wrote a letter to Mills stating that the patient had evolved to the point of expressing himself in complete sentences of considerable length that were formed of his own volition. Thus, it would appear that response to treatment had been quite positive. In the published discussion that followed the presentation of this and other cases, however, a Dr. Burr from Philadelphia noted that "it is very hard for us to say how much of the improvement is due to education and how much is due to the natural course of events" (p. 1948). This may be the first record of what is a continuing skepticism regarding the efficacy of aphasia therapy—a skepticism later directed towards the work of speech-language pathologists as our field developed and treatment of aphasia became our purview.

Dr. Weisenburg, who participated in the retraining of Mills' agrammatic patient, went on to coauthor with the psychologist Katherine McBride, the 1935 text *Aphasia: A Clinical and Psychological Study,* in which they introduced the terms "expressive" and "receptive" aphasia. The study, which was carried out in 1929, was supported by a grant from the Commonwealth Fund. Patients studied were given a battery of language and cognitive tests and followed longitudinally in a search for recovery patterns. Some received treatment, including a 45-year-old woman (Case 24) with chronic hypertension who had a stroke during gynecologic surgery. She was examined 2 weeks after onset, then remained without training or any other examination for 7 months, when she was retested. She then began treatment at the rate of 1 or 2 hours a week with home practice and was retested after 6 and then 12 months of treatment. Thus, four data points were obtained: 2 weeks post-onset, after 7 months with no treatment, after 6 months of treatment, and after 6 more months of treatment. All test results were displayed in a graph that showed "there had been far more improvement" (p. 395) during the first 6 months of treatment than the first 7 months postonset. Test results on the third and fourth exams clustered around her educational level. Thus, Weisenburg and McBride appear to have been the first to establish patient performance baselines and use repeated dependent test measures to determine the effects of aphasia therapy. Their description of the therapy techniques employed are somewhat scant, however.

For a detailed description of aphasia treatment methods and "on-line" responses to these methods we can turn back to a paper published in 1905 by Shepherd Ivory Franz, a pathophysiologist. One month after onset of severe aphasia, a 57-year-old man was erroneously taken to a hospital for the insane where Franz was working. Franz then began to systematically teach the man the names of 10 familiar colors, the numbers 1–10, a short stanza of poetry, the Lord's Prayer, and the German equivalents of a few common English words. An example of his methods follows. In training color naming, Franz showed the patient color cards one at a time and asked him to name them. If he named the color correctly he was told "correct," if not, he was told "wrong" and given two more tries to name before being given the name and asked to repeat it. If the patient said he did not know the name after the first trial, the name was given to him immediately. Results were recorded in tables displaying session dates, percentage of correct answers, number of experiments, number of mistakes in naming each color, and frequency of wrong word production based on a naming test given at the beginning of each session. The patient improved slowly until he could list the 10 color names without seeing the cards. The return of skills was gradual and this led Franz to conjecture that recovery did not occur solely because old brain paths were being reopened but rather because new connections were being made. He spoke of the "vicarious" function of the cerebrum, in which one part or one hemisphere may take up the lost functions of another part or side.

Franz continued his study of aphasia and in 1924 published an 80-page paper in which he described two types of re-education experiments. The first was directed specifically at rehabilitation with the purpose of the second to determine the course of improvement under controlled experimental conditions where the results could be recorded and tabulated. This paper may be the most detailed account of aphasia retraining methods ever published and includes descriptions of cases treated at 3 years and 6 years postonset. Among Franz's conclusions is that patients who appear to have similar patterns of aphasia are likely to show individual differences on close examination. He went on to say that "accurate records of re-education endeavors must be kept in order to adapt the procedure to individual needs" (p. 429).

What is clear from these early aphasia treatment cases is that therapy often extended over many months and even years. In her 1918 paper, Bumgardner, a speech remediation specialist, described a man who was treated for 160 weeks with six 1½-hour lessons a week. Prior to beginning therapy with her, this man had been unable to speak for 3 years. With treatment, he "relearned sufficient language to enable him to speak spontaneously and correctly almost any word he desires, and sometimes perfectly correct language to express his thoughts" (p. 154). Bumgardner ends her paper with the following impassioned statement:

No one who has not endured three years of silence without even one word with which to voice his emotion can estimate the joy of a man who after striving faithfully at least is rewarded by speaking distinctly and joining freely into conversation with his friends, even though his language scope is limited. (p. 154)

Another poignant case serves to underscore Bumgardner's observation. In 1933, Singer and Low, two physicians from London and Chicago, respectively, reported on a case they treated together over a number of years. In 1904, a 39-year-old woman had a stroke after giving birth. She had right hemiplegia and aphasia, which limited her speech to the stereotypic utterance "o-de-dar." She was sent to a nursing home. When seen in spring 1906 (2 years later), she was unable to walk and produced only her verbal stereotypy, although she seemed to understand everything that was said to her. Not surprisingly, she was greatly frustrated. Dr. Low began her aphasia therapy by teaching her the "b" sound through blowing and then combining the "b" with "ee" to say "bee," with "o" for "bow," and with "ar" for "bar." He then taught her husband to work with her daily in teaching combinations of consonant and vowel sounds, later adding final consonants for words such as bed, book, pin, cup and progressing to two-syllable words. At the same time, she practiced walking. Two years later, she was able to travel to England where she went under the care of Dr. Singer. When she returned to the United States, she had a useful vocabulary of about 500 words, and was able to do household duties such as cooking, although she never regained right hand function. She learned to make grocery lists, participate in church affairs, and oversee her daughter's education. She died in November 1929, having lived an active life in the 23 years after leaving the nursing home. Postmortem examination of her brain showed a large cavity in the left second and third frontal convolutions, with sparing of the temporal lobe and right hemisphere. Given the total destruction of language zones subserving speech output, one might conjecture that the intact right hemisphere (as suggested by Mills in 1904) was recruited in learning those 500 words that allowed her to communicate and participate in life so successfully.

These early aphasia treatment cases reflect the lack of knowledge about the nuances of this complex disorder; but following World War II, with many wounded soldiers returning to military hospitals, aphasia came under closer scrutiny. The return of scores of brain-damaged soldiers in Russia allowed the neuropsychologist Alexander Luria to study and treat aphasia. In a series of case studies (Luria, 1970), he described his rationales and methods for treating various forms of aphasia. For example, he discussed patients with agrammatism who were able to comprehend relatively complex logico-grammatical relationships, but produced little more than nouns in their own speech. He said such patients are unable to create the inner dynamic schema for any type of grammatical, predicative statement. He believed that restoration of their expressive speech could be achieved by substituting external aids for the missing inner schema. Luria described an agrammatic patient who, as a basis for making predicative statements, was taught that any statement involving a single word was incomplete. He then was given instructions that forced him to attach a verb or adjective to every object mentioned. Luria thought that external schemata used must represent the relationships between objects and must lead to conscious awareness of the grammatical rules adhered to in normal speech. He made diagrams (some of which are displayed in his text) that made use of pictures and abstract symbols for constructing sentences. In concluding his remarks on aphasia therapy, he stated that, "A consciously directed, systematic course of retraining is the only method of compensating for a defect arising from primary brain damage. By reorganizing the disturbed function it is possible to restore activities which once appeared hopelessly lost" (p. 458).

Luria's work with aphasia was highly sophisticated for its time (and arguably even for the present time), but during the 1960s the fields of linguistics and psycholinguistics expanded enormously and the mysteries of language came under close scrutiny. In England, speech pathologist F. M. Hatfield began applying knowledge from these fields to the treatment of aphasia. In her 1972 paper, "Looking for Help from Linguistics," she stressed the importance of determining which levels of language are disturbed in a given aphasia case, whether any rules are operating within the deviant speech, whether language competency or only performance is impaired, and whether the patient is having difficulty in finding or combining words. At the same time, Hatfield acknowledged the limitations of a linguistic approach to aphasia therapy. In treating patients, she said that linguistic principles could not account for some errors that seem to have instead resulted from such factors as perseveration, fatigue, inattention, motivation, or poor relevance of the material for the patient. We are well aware today that these factors must be attended to, if any aphasia treatment program is to be carried out successfully.

II. CURRENT CASE STUDIES

Since the early 1970s there has been an explosion of literature pertaining to treatment of aphasia and many additional case studies can be found in scientific journals and books. These reports include a large number of patients whose treatment has been couched in methodologically rigorous single-subject experimental treatment designs and detailed descriptions of the treatment methods. Regardless of their varied treatment formats, however, roots for virtually all of the treatment methods currently employed can be traced to earlier publications, only a few of which have been mentioned here. From these roots a substantial tree of knowledge has grown and this tree reaches out to allied fields for its continued nourishment. The chapters in this book make the point clear. Here one finds sophisticated single-subject methodology, as well as theoretical advances in linguistics, interpersonal communication, and cognitive psychology all applied to the treatment process. Although the management approaches of each author are diverse, each describes the considerations that guided their clinical approaches. And, while acknowledging the roots of their methods, they each describe the individualistic and principled steps they use to strengthen these methods. This is how a profession advances.

Some authors in this volume break new ground in terms of the cases they report. Relatively few workers have reported specifically on reading problems, even fewer on the problems involved in alexia without agraphia. Beeson and Gonzalez-Rothi (and colleagues) describe their work with individuals who have such reading impairments. Both patients are letter-by-letter readers. Both clinical reports invoke processing models to establish rationales for treatment, acknowledging thereby the growing role that such models are beginning to play in the development of treatment approaches. And then their case reports diverge. Treatments for each patient differed, and one was more successful than the other. For Beeson's more successful case, her original model provided her with explicit notions about how to modify it for even more effective utilization. For Gonzalez-Rothi and colleagues, a different challenge arose. They use their model to provide clues for why their treatment did not work. In the process, they raise several very pertinent clinical questions and provide a number of interesting alternatives. Finally, both Beeson and Gonzalez-Rothi and colleagues come to a similar conclusion: We need to know why methods work with some patients and not others. In obtaining this information, we obviously must study patients who respond well to our methods. Looking at what fails to work is often equally, if not more, instructive. Both are important to determining the best match between clinical approaches and patients.

Berndt and Mitchum and Thompson describe far more commonly encountered patients—agrammatic speakers with Broca's aphasia. Once again, rationales are clearly spelled out. Both case studies focus on the core role of verbs and verb argument structures for understanding the problems central to agrammatic speech. Berndt and Mitchum focused on their patient's difficulty with sentence comprehension, while Thompson focused on sentence production. Both cases made demonstrable improvement as the result of attention to very different aspects of their common problems. In Berndt and Mitchum's case, generalization to untrained sentence comprehension was obtained. Thompson also reports generalization to untrained sentences and to the increased use of verbs and verb argument structures in speech production. These reports are linked by another very important concept for aphasia rehabilitation. Even in patients who have what appear to be very similar profiles, different aspects of their problems can be profitably treated. Thus, there is no single "treatment for Broca's aphasia patients" (or for any other type). Instead, there are various treatments, each having highly specific and appropriate outcomes. The wise clinician has a variety of clinical approaches available and can match them, not only with a language problem at hand, but with the client who is most likely to profit from them.

The cases of Helm-Estabrooks and Lyon present even greater contrast. Helm-Estabrooks chose to focus her work on neuropsychological processes that underlie the linguistic aspects of aphasia. She cogently argues that such work was necessary for her patient to reestablish his ability to connect with the world of language. At the other end of the therapy continuum, Lyon assisted a couple who must deal with the devastating effects of aphasia. His goal for treatment was to improve psychosocial functioning. To accomplish this, the couple had to change spousal roles and find ways to reestablish interactive patterns. Some very important observations link the work of Helm-Estabrooks and Lyon. Their combined message is that the aphasia treatment need not be limited to direct manipulation of language, but, instead, can range from work with underlying neuropsychology processes to helping patients and families live successfully with aphasia.

The chapters of Wertz and Holland can arguably be linked as well. They are at different ends of yet another continuum—in their cases, the frequency of occurrence of a problem. Wertz describes a very common problem in aphasia and Holland describes a very unusual one. Wertz' case is one that has perplexed clinicians often as they have tried to determine effective treatment strategies and the order in which the treatments should be presented. He describes a case of aphasia, accompanied by not one, but two, apraxias—one of speech and the other of phonation. Holland describes a problem that might have been incompletely or inaccurately diagnosed in the absence of detailed, highly personalized clinical evaluation. Both Wertz and Holland provide detailed analyses of what went into their thinking as they devised their approaches to diagnosis and treatment. These reports illustrate that careful and detailed therapy planning almost always pays off.

And finally, there is Frattali's contribution. She describes the environment of treatment delivery as we move into the next century. She then provides an analysis of the case studies in this book—a report card on how these cases might fit into changing context for aphasia treatment. Frattali describes a pathway that aphasia treatment may take in the future. She conveys that aphasia treatment may be limited to a few sessions and, therefore, will need to become more streamlined. At the same time she stresses the continuing need for individual case reports.

Case reports have played a strong role in our professional history and they should continue to do so in the future. We hope that this book will be a model for others to follow in reporting what they have done to bring about positive changes in their patients. We also hope that some of the ideas presented here will be useful to clinicians in their daily clinical practice.

III. ACKNOWLEDGMENTS

This work was supported, in part, by the National Institute for Deafness and Communication Disorders Grant No. DC1409 to the National Center for Neurogenic Communication Disorders at the University of Arizona.

IV. REFERENCES

Broadbent, D. (1979). A case of peculiar affection of speech, with commentary. *Brain, 1,* 484–503.

Broca, P. (1865). Sur la faculté du langage articulé. *Bulletin de la Société d'Antropologie, 6,* 337–393.

Bumgardner, A. C. (1918). A victim of aphasia regains speech through instruction with the oral method. *Volta Review, 20,* 152–155.

Franz, S. I. (1905). The reeducation of an aphasic. *Journal of Philosophy, Psychology and Scientific Methods, 2*(22), 589–597.

Franz, S. I. (1924). Studies in re-education: The aphasias. *Journal of Comparative Psychology, 4,* 349–429.

Hatfield, F. M. (1972). Looking for help from linguistics. *British Journal of Communication Disorders, 7*(1), 64–81.

Luria, A. R. (1970). *Traumatic aphasia: Its syndromes, psychology, and treatment.* The Hague: Mouton.

Mills, C. K. (1880, May). Clinical lectures. *The Medical Bulletin,* Philadelphia, 23–28.

Mills, C. K. (1904). Treatment of aphasia by training. *Journal of the American Medical Association, 43,* 1940–1949.

Singer, H. D., & Low, A. A. (1933). The brain in a case of motor aphasia in which improvement occurred with training. *Archives of Neurology and Psychiatry, 29,* 162–165.

Weisenburg, T., & McBride, K. E. (1935). *Aphasia: A clinical and psychological study.* New York: Hafner Publishing Co.

Wyllie, J. (1894). *The disorders of speech.* Edinburgh: Oliver and Boyd.

CHAPTER

2

A Case of Aphasia, Apraxia of Speech, and Apraxia of Phonation

ROBERT T. WERTZ, Ph.D.

I. BACKGROUND

Life is not fair for those who suffer neurogenic communication disorders. Conditions brought about by neurological chance may shatter speech and language. Not only can a disorder exist, but also disorders may coexist.

A. The Dilemma of Definitions

Those who manage neurogenic communication disorders may not employ the same nosology. They may differ in what they call the same thing and in what they call different things. That is okay. Controversy does not necessarily demean us. It can elevate us.

Patients who suffer apraxia of speech wear masks, which appear aphasic, yet conspire with dysarthria. The apraxia of the speech patient's disguise may be so effective that some authors (Martin, 1974) deny the disorder exists. Others have written chapters (Duffy, 1995; Rosenbek, 1985) and books (Square-Storer, 1989; Wertz, LaPointe, & Rosenbek, 1984) about it. Some (Goodglass & Kaplan, 1983) submerge the disorder in aphasia: typically, Broca's aphasia. Others (Darley, 1982) believe the signs are sufficiently different to justify a name—apraxia of speech. However, most are good observers. And, regardless of their theoretical preferences, all can identify the salient signs that some call apraxia of speech.

1. **Aphasia.** For me, this is an impairment due to acquired damage of the central nervous system of the ability to comprehend and formulate language; a multimodality disorder represented by a variety of impairments in auditory comprehension, reading, oral-expressive language, and writing; that cannot be explained by dementia, sensory loss, or motor dysfunction (Rosenbek, LaPointe, & Wertz, 1989).

2. **Apraxia of Speech.** For me, this is a neurogenic speech disorder resulting from sensorimotor impairment of the capacity to program and execute in coordinated and normally timed sequences, the positioning of the speech musculature for the volitional production of speech sounds with loss or impairment of phonologic rules not being adequate to explain the observed pattern of deviant speech— nor is the disturbance attributable to weakened or misdirected actions of specific muscle groups (Wertz et al., 1984).

   Salient signs of apraxia of speech are: effortful, trial-and-error, groping articulatory movements, and attempts at self-correction; dysprosody unrelieved by extended periods of normal rhythm, stress, and intonation; articulatory inconsistency on repeated productions of the same utterance; and obvious difficulty initiating utterances.

3. **Apraxia of Phonation.** For me, this is an inability to program volitionally the initiation and/or maintenance of phonation in the absence of significant laryngeal paralysis. Simpson and Clark (1989) call this condition apractic mutism. Lebrun (1990) suggests it is a part of motor aphasia. Nevertheless, apraxia of phonation, as used here, is the inability to produce sound volitionally in the absence of laryngeal paralysis. The patient with apraxia of phonation will produce sound nonvolitionally, for example by throat clearing,

coughing, and laughing. On voluntary attempts to produce sound, the patient typically emits a rush of air through abducted vocal folds.

B. Rationale for Treatment

1. **Treating Aphasia.** Probably, there are as many methods for treating aphasia as there are clinicians treating it. A general dichotomy for treatment is restoration of language (specific techniques for restoring auditory comprehension, reading, oral-expressive language [phonology, semantics, and syntax], and writing) versus restoration of communication (prompting the use of any means or combination of means [gesturing, writing, drawing, speaking] to convey and receive information for achieving transactions [imparting specific information] or interactions ["hanging out"]).

2. **Treating Apraxia of Speech.** Methods will vary. However, most are designed to facilitate or reorganize impaired motor speech programming, increasing the probability of producing intended phonemes and the sequencing of phonemes in intelligible utterances. Generally, this is accomplished through motor speech drill: repetitive attempts that require the apraxic person to know the necessary articulatory movements to produce specific sounds and plan, execute, and evaluate the production.

3. **Treating Apraxia of Phonation.** Once it is established that the laryngeal mechanism is capable of producing phonation—absence of significant paralysis and evidence of adequate laryngeal closure in nonvolitional activities (throat clearing, coughing, laughing)— treatment is focused on developing consistent, reliable voicing. The literature for treating apraxia of phonation is sparse. Dworkin and Abkarian (1996) suggest employing a hierarchy of stimuli—isolated vowels, three-vowel sequences, and alternating vowel and glottal [h] consonant sequences (i.e., a-h-a-h-a-h, etc.). Simpson and Clark (1989) list a variety of techniques, including giving the patient a "running start" with sentence completion or "close" techniques ["Wind the _____" (watch)]; rote productions: counting, singing, or reciting nursery rhymes; melodic intonation therapy (Albert, Sparks, & Helm, 1973); and vegetative responses: grunting by pushing against physical resistance.

4. **Treatment for Coexisting Disorders.** When disorders coexist, the clinician typically makes one of three choices: treat one disorder

exclusively, treat each disorder separately but simultaneously, or select a single treatment that may provide management for all disorders simultaneously. Rationale for the first approach might be to select and treat the disorder that is most disruptive to communication and that is expected to resolve most rapidly with the least time and effort. Additional rationale for this choice might be to treat the disorder that must resolve before treatment of the other disorder or disorders can be treated. For example, if severe apraxia of speech coexists with severe aphasia, one usually opts to treat the aphasia until sufficient oral-expressive production is present to permit focusing treatment for the apraxia of speech. The second approach—separate but simultaneous treatment—would involve dividing the treatment time into tasks designed to improve each of the patient's disorders, for example, 15 minutes on apraxia of phonation, 15 minutes on apraxia of speech, and 30 minutes on aphasia. The third option, simultaneous treatment of all disorders with a single method, for example, melodic intonation therapy, may stimulate voicing for the apraxia of phonation, improve articulation through drill for the apraxia of speech, and provide semantics and syntax through repetition of the phrase stimuli for the aphasia. In the absence of empirical evidence to support one method over another, clinicians make a choice. The patient's performance will indicate whether the choice was correct. Patients are good at that.

II. THE PATIENT

A. Biography

D. M., "Doug," was a 37-year-old, white male who resided in a small, Northern California city. He had graduated from high school, spent 2 years in a variety of jobs in the construction business, completed a 3-year tour of duty in the Army, returned home, and re-entered the construction trade as a carpenter. Doug had never married and, except for his military service, always lived in the family home with his widowed mother. Two older brothers lived nearby with their families. Doug filled his days with work and his evenings "running" with high school buddies and "guys from the job," or watching TV. His passions were his 1956 Chevy BelAire and watching vintage war movies. He smoked two packs a day, retired a six-pack of beer on weeknights, and doubled that consumption on weekends. His mother reported that Doug was a "good boy" but "lacked ambition."

B. Medical History

Doug's last contact with doctors had been at age 23, when he received a discharge physical from the Army. There was no history of stroke in his immediate family. His father died of lung cancer at age 52. Maternal and paternal grandparents, according to Doug's mother, died in their early 70s, "probably of old age."

Approximately 1 month before we met, Doug's mother realized he had not "left for work." She found him in bed, "unable to talk and paralyzed on his right side." A trip to the local hospital resulted in a diagnosis of "stroke" with subsequent "right hemiplegia and expressive aphasia." After a 1-week stay, he was discharged home to the care of his mother. After 2 weeks at home, Doug's persisting right hemiplegia, inability to communicate, mother's work schedule, and lack of rehabilitation facilities in the community resulted in his transfer to our Veterans Administration Medical Center, 150 miles south of his home.

A neurological evaluation at 3-weeks postonset revealed a large, left hemisphere infarct in the middle cerebral artery distribution. Figure 2–1, a computerized reconstruction of Doug's CT scan, indicates the lesion was cortical and subcortical and involved the left frontal, temporal, and parietal areas and extended into the insula. Visual acuity was 20/30 in each eye, and there were no field abnormalities, nystagmus, extraocular movement, or gaze impairment. A dense, right hemiplegia was present, with slightly more impairment in the upper extremity. A "moderate" right, lower facial weakness was noted. A mental status examination revealed no mood abnormalities or significant intellectual impairment. The neurologist concluded that Doug had suffered a "thrombosis of the left middle cerebral artery with right hemiparesis and predominately expressive aphasia." Subsequent hearing screening indicated an estimated 10 dB speech reception threshold bilaterally.

III. APPRAISAL

A. Methods

During the 3rd week postonset, an appraisal of speech, voice, and language was conducted. A motor speech evaluation (Wertz et al., 1984) provided an indication of the presence or absence of apraxia of speech and/or dysarthria and, if present, the severity of each. Voice was appraised perceptually in the motor speech evaluation and a consultation

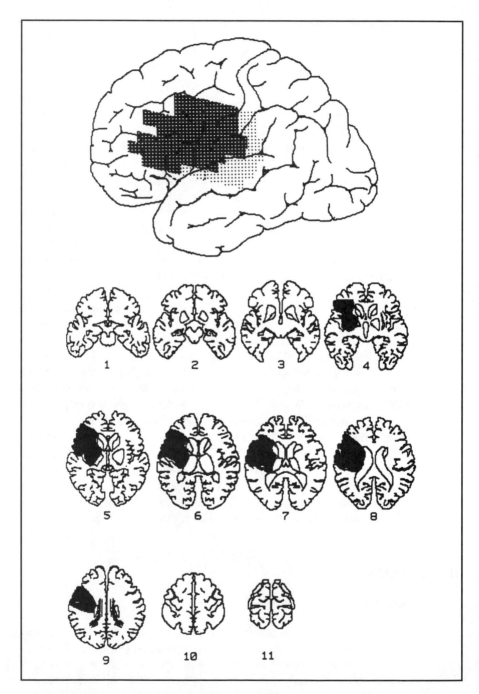

Figure 2–1. Computerized reconstruction of CT scan at 3 weeks postonset.

by otolaryngology was requested. Appraisal of language impairment included administering the *Porch Index of Communicative Ability* (PICA) (Porch, 1967); *Boston Diagnostic Aphasia Examination* (BDAE) (Goodglass & Kaplan, 1983); aphasia quotient (AQ) subtests in the *Western Aphasia Battery* (WAB) (Kertesz, 1982); and the *Token Test* (Spreen & Benton, 1969). Appraisal of communicative disability was done by administering the *Communicative Abilities in Daily Living* (CADL) (Holland, 1980).

B. Results

Doug's performance on the appraisal battery is shown in Table 2–1.

1. **Speech.** The motor speech evaluation revealed a probable "severe" apraxia of speech: "7" on a 7-point scale, where "1" indicates normal. "Probable" was used, because Doug produced random articulatory movements and only a rush of air through abducted vocal folds. Attempts to produce vowels revealed articulatory groping, starts, stops, and eventually a steady stream of unphonated air. Attempts to produce repeated monosyllables—pʌ, tʌ, and kʌ—revealed the same articulatory behaviors, however productions were interrupted and produced in segments. Similarly, attempts to repeat mono- and polysyllabic words indicated articulatory groping, attempts at self-correction, and on repeated attempts of the same utterance, articulatory inconsistency. If dysarthria was present, it was mild: "2" on the 7-point scale. Voiceless consonants were reasonably crisp, but they were substitutions for the requested sounds.

Table 2–1. Performance on appraisal measures pretreatment, 3 weeks, postonset

Measure	Performance
PICA	
Overall	33rd %ile
Gestural	54th %ile
Verbal	18th %ile
Graphic	35th %ile
WAB AQ	16.60
Token Test Total Score	112
CADL Total Score	62
Apraxia of Speech Rating	7

Oral-nonverbal apraxia (buccal-facial apraxia) was present. Doug was unable to produce nonspeech tongue, lip, jaw, and laryngeal movements, for example, tongue protrusion and elevation, blowing, smiling, mouth opening, throat clearing, and coughing consistently or reliably, on command or by imitation. However, many of these movements were present nonvolitionally, for example, lip licking and throat clearing. No drooling or pooling of saliva was observed and Doug had no difficulty swallowing.

Evaluation of limb praxis, by command and imitation, indicated good gestures, both simple: "show me okay" and complex: "pretend to unlock a door and open it."

2. **Voice.** All volitional attempts at vocalization evoked unphonated rushes of air. However, Doug indicated he could approximate his vocal folds by nonvolitional throat clearing and coughing. Moreover, he produced sound following my inane attempts to get him to laugh: "One way to get your vocal cords together is for me to choke you." The otolaryngology consultation indicated no significant vocal fold paralysis during indirect laryngoscopy; however, movement was observed primarily on gag and nonvolitional throat clearing and coughing.

3. **Language.** Figure 2–2 indicates Doug's performance on the PICA. He was at the 33rd overall percentile, and gestural and graphic performance, although impaired, was superior to verbal performance. Auditory comprehension, subtests VI and X, indicated a few delays for one-step commands. Reading, subtests V and VII, was correct but incomplete: Nouns and verbs were read, but prepositions of place were ignored. Visual matching, subtests VIII and XI, was prompt and correct. Pantomimic ability, subtests II and III, was correct but incomplete. Writing, subtests A–D, was nonfunctional, however he could copy words and geometric shapes, subtests E and F, in a correct but distorted, delayed, and incomplete manner. All verbal tasks, subtests I, IV, IX, and XII, were attempted but, eventually, rejected. The Token Test supported and expanded the PICA auditory subtest performance. Doug scored 112 out of the possible 163. Errors clustered on the longer and more complex auditory commands.

Figure 2–3 shows Doug's profile of speech characteristics on the BDAE. Melodic line, phrase length, articulatory agility, and grammatical form were either sparse or absent. There were no paraphasias in running speech, because there was no running speech.

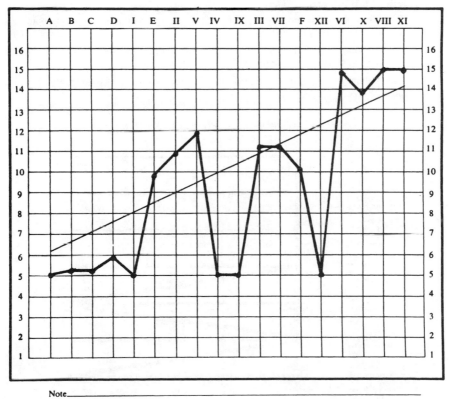

Figure 2–2. PICA ranked response summary at 3 weeks postonset.

Patient's Name ___D.M.___   Date of rating _8/26/83_

Rated by ___RTW___

<u>APHASIA SEVERITY RATING SCALE</u>

0. No usable speech or auditory comprehension.

(1) All communication is through fragmentary expression; great need for inference, questioning, and guessing by the listener. The range of information that can be exchanged is limited, and the listener carries the burden of communication.

2. Conversation about familiar subjects is possible with help from the listener. There are frequent failures to convey the idea, but patient shares the burden of communication with the examiner.

3. The patient can discuss <u>almost all everyday problems</u> with little or no assistance. Reduction of speech and/or comprehension, however, makes conversation about certain material difficult or impossible.

4. Some obvious loss of fluency in speech or facility of comprehension, without significant limitation on ideas expressed or form of expression.

5. Minimal discernible speech handicaps; patient may have subjective difficulties that are not apparent to listener.

RATING SCALE PROFILE OF SPEECH CHARACTERISTICS

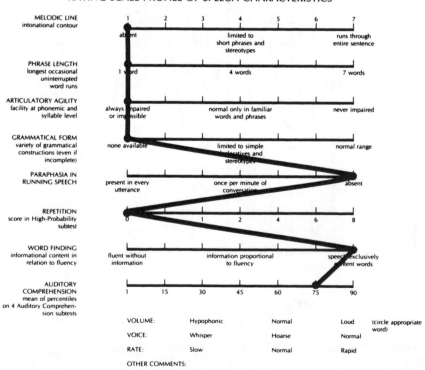

Apraxia of phonation

Figure 2–3. BDAE rating scale profile of speech characteristics at 3 weeks postonset.

Similarly, repetition was absent. Word finding was rated "exclusively content words," except he produced no words. And, auditory comprehension was at the 75th percentile. His severity rating was "1," and his profile was consistent with Broca's aphasia. The WAB AQ was 16.60 out of the possible 100. His points came, exclusively, from the auditory comprehension subtests. The WAB classification also indicated Broca's aphasia.

CADL performance was 62 out of the possible 136. Doug communicated better than he talked. With repetitions, he used gestural, written, and drawing responses to indicate his functional communication, though impaired, was not too shabby.

IV. DIAGNOSIS

A. Aphasia

Doug's performance on the PICA, BDAE, WAB, and Token Test was consistent with my definition of aphasia: a general language deficit crossing all communicative modalities—auditory comprehension, reading, oral-expressive language, and writing. The presence of apraxia of speech and apraxia of phonation complicated my view of oral-expressive language impairment because of Doug's paucity of production. However, his limited oral-expressive productions suggested the presence of significant semantic and syntactic impairment. Doug's aphasia was moderately severe even after factoring out his apraxia of speech and apraxia of phonation. His PICA percentiles were 33rd overall, 54th gestural, 18th verbal, and 35th graphic. Auditory comprehension was significantly impaired—54th percentile on the PICA and 69% correct on the Token Test. Similarly, reading was impaired—45th percentile on the PICA. Doug's functional communication, as indicated by his CADL performance, was poor—62 out of the possible 136. However, he performed above the mean (54.23) for Broca's aphasic patients in Holland's (1980) standardization sample.

B. Apraxia of Speech

Doug's paucity of verbal production made a diagnosis of apraxia of speech difficult. Nevertheless, he appeared to meet my definition: impaired ability to program and execute volitional production of speech sounds that could not be explained by the presence of significant dysarthria. His attempts at production were effortful: He groped for articulatory positions, he attempted to correct his inadequate productions, he had particular difficulty initiating utterances, and he displayed articulatory inconsistency on repeated productions of the same utterances. Such is the behavior I call apraxia of speech. So, I said it was most severe: "7" on the 7-point severity scale.

C. Apraxia of Phonation

To apply the label apraxia of phonation, one must demonstrate an inability to program volitional production and maintenance of phonation in the absence of significant laryngeal paralysis. Doug's effortful attempts to produce sound resulted in unvocalized rushes of air. His phonation during nonvolitional laughing and good vocal fold closure during nonvolitional coughing and throat clearing implied the absence of laryngeal paralysis. Confirmation of no significant laryngeal paralysis by otolaryngology made me suspect I had caught myself a case of apraxia of phonation.

V. PROGNOSIS

A. Prognostic Methods

Predicting a future for aphasic people is not precise. Ability to do the same for people with apraxia of speech is worse. And, for those with apraxia of phonation, prognostic precision is nil. However, "Will I improve and how much?" are the most important questions patients ask, and we attempt to provide answers. Our methods include experience with prognostic variables—age, severity, size of lesion, health status, and so on—and behavioral profiles generated by a few standardized measures, for example, PICA high overall prediction (HOAP and HOAP slopes).

B. Expected Outcome

1. **Language Impairment.** Applying prognostic variables to Doug was enigmatic. He was young, healthy, and close to onset; all favorable signs for improvement. However, his lesion was large; a bad sign. And, he was moderately aphasic; a neutral sign. Using the PICA HOAP slopes, I predicted his 33rd percentile overall performance at approximately 1 month postonset should improve to the 43rd percentile at 3 months postonset and the 60th percentile at 6 months postonset. These predictions, however, were tempered by his apraxia of phonation and apraxia of speech.

2. **Language Disability.** To predict improvement in functional communication, we use our experience, hunches, and hopes. Specifi-

cally, we ask: can and how willing is the patient to employ all available means to communicate—attention, facial expression, gesturing, drawing, and *use* of residual auditory comprehension, reading, oral-expressive language, and writing. Those who can and are willing to employ alternatives become better functional communicators. Those who are not do not. Equally important is the willingness of those in the patient's environment to encourage and employ alternatives to traditional communication. I knew little about those in Doug's environment. But, I observed he attended closely and utilized facial expression, gestures, drawing, and attempts at writing to communicate. Because he did all of these without being taught or asked, I predicted his functional communication would improve with direction, additional strategies, and practice.

3. **Apraxia of Speech.** Wertz et al. (1984) wrote, "Prognosis [for apraxia of speech] is an exercise in augury" (p. 132). A trip to the literature does not help. Vignolo (1964) said, "anarthria has a significant retarding effect on recovery of expression" (p. 367). However, Mohr (1980) observed, "A person whose infarction is confined to Broca's area experiences an initial period of mutism with some disturbance in language function, followed quickly thereafter by the emergence of speech . . . taking the form of speech dysprosody or speech dyspraxia" (p. 2–3).

What we know about the future for people with apraxia of speech has been teased, for the most part, from what we know about prognosis for aphasia. I (Wertz, 1984) found no significant relationships between initial severity of apraxia of speech or change in apraxia of speech with age or education. Initial severity was related significantly with improvement in apraxia of speech—more severely affected patients improved less. Some (Butfield, 1958; Vignolo, 1964; Webb & Love, 1974) caution that the presence of oral, nonverbal apraxia will interfere with improvement in apraxia of speech. Others (Bowman, Hodson, & Simpson, 1980; De Renzi, Pieczuro, & Vignolo, 1966; LaPointe & Wertz, 1974) found no significant relationship between severity of oral, nonverbal apraxia and severity of apraxia of speech.

Doug's apraxia of speech was severe—"7" on the 1–7 rating scale. In addition, it was complicated by the presence of aphasia, apraxia of phonation, and oral-nonverbal apraxia. If we believe the literature, Doug's combination of disorders forecasted a bleak future for improvement in his apraxia of speech. Searching for some sunshine in the cloudy forecast, I seized on his age (young) and time postonset (short). Even these restricted prognostic adjectives to "poor" or "guarded."

4. **Apraxia of Phonation.** Seeking predictors of improvement in apraxia of phonation makes those for aphasia and apraxia of speech seem abundant. Simpson and Clark (1989), summarizing the meager literature on apractic mutism, concluded that the condition is usually transient and improves rapidly with no intervention. However, in some patients, muteness persists and requires intervention. Rosenbek (1985) suggested that apraxia of phonation that persists for a few days is predictive of a poor prognosis for its improvement. Vignolo (1964) agrees, however he extends the period to 2 months. Wertz et al. (1984) concluded that, "mutism that persists is likely to be mutism that will continue to persist" (p. 144).

Nevertheless, my experience had been that apraxia of phonation seldom persisted, and I thought I had some clinical magic that could produce phonation quickly and consistently in the mutest of the mute. Thus, I speculated Doug would be phonating, and our time together would be spent on rolling back his aphasia and apraxia of speech. Beware speculation!

VI. FOCUSING THE TREATMENT

Doug was available to spend an hour a day with me, 5 days a week, for at least a month. Initially, I elected to attack two of his problems—apraxia of phonation and aphasia—simultaneously, but separately. If one—apraxia of phonation—could be solved, it would be dropped from the treatment agenda and replaced by an assault on Doug's apraxia of speech. Therefore, I divided our efforts into producing sound—eliminate the apraxia of phonation; developing functional communication through gesture, writing, and drawing; and, once reliable phonation was obtained, attacking his apraxia of speech with motor speech drill. Each hour would be divided, not necessarily equally, into these efforts. Traditional? Of course! Tradition is a good reason for carrying on when there are so many reasons not to.

A. Obtaining Phonation

My experience dictated that phonation could be achieved rapidly in folks with apraxia of phonation by laying on the hands. I place my hand on the patient's abdominal area, ask him or her to take a breath, and to exhale slowly. About halfway through the exhalation, I apply a strong push against the patient's abdomen. This should be firm, not violent.

Patients with apraxia of phonation typically do what you and I would do if we were "jabbed" in the belly during exhalation. They lock their vocal folds and produce a strong, audible "unhhh!" A patient's response to producing voice on volitional exhalation is typically surprise—both from being punched in the stomach and from producing voice. Quickly, this is followed by volitional voice production, perhaps to avoid repeated blows to the belly, and, perhaps, from the realization that he or she can produce voice. I forget where I learned this magic, but I suspect it was among the many useful things Tom Hixon taught me about managing respiration and phonation in motor speech disorders.

My plan was to have Doug lock his vocal folds and produce sound when coaxed by my manual manipulation. The goal was to obtain reliable and acceptable phonation on vowels and ensure phonation generalized to attempts at other productions. Once this was obtained, our work on Doug's apraxia of phonation would be done, and we would see what the noise he would be making told us about his apraxia of speech and how it could be mended.

B. Obtaining Communication

A decision was necessary regarding the focus of communication therapy. Should it emphasize restoring language—auditory comprehension, reading, oral-expressive language, and writing; emphasize communication—receiving and imparting information by any means available; or should it be a combination of the two? I, with agreement from Doug, elected the middle road—emphasize communication.

My rationale for this decision was based on Doug's strengths and weaknesses. His auditory comprehension and reading were adequate. His oral-expressive language was submerged in a morass of apraxia of phonation and apraxia of speech. Until these improved, increased oral-expressive language would be imprisoned behind an unscaleable wall of motor speech disorder. Doug's propositional writing was nonfunctional, but he could get a start on some words—by producing the initial letters accurately. And he would, with coaxing, supplement his incomplete, but accurate, gestures with drawing. Finally, he had developed the idea that communicating without speech was okay. So, emphasis was placed on communication, and it included equal parts of what people do when they do that—transaction and interaction.

1. **Transaction.** For me, transaction requires imparting specific information: answering the question, "Who called?" and conveying how to get to Tootsie's Orchard Lounge. I am surprised how seldom

we transact. However, when transaction is required, there is no substitute. But, there are ways to transact that do not require speech.

Our work on Doug's ability to impart specific information included first, deciding what kinds of specific information he needed to impart in his environment, the rehabilitation ward and program, and his future environment, home. Doug was the source of this information, and my obtaining it provided a pragmatic context for training him to utilize the means he had available to impart it. He had adequate auditory comprehension and the reading ability to understand my questions; could request repeats, elaborations, and alternatives when he didn't understand; could utilize gesture, including pantomime and pointing to a variety of resource media (newspapers, magazines, maps, lists, schedules, etc.); could provide written responses within his resources, including correction and rejection of his written errors (rejecting the "W" he wrote for the first letter of his home town when it began with a "U"); and could supplement his gestures and writing by drawing pictures.

After the information to be transacted was identified, Doug required little training in how to impart it. He had learned that when we collected what we thought he needed to convey. The list was kept open, and a part of each treatment session was spent in adding to it. I alerted those in his environment—other therapists, nurses, physicians, wardmates—how Doug communicated and how to assist him in doing that.

2. **Interaction.** For me, interaction requires keeping up one's side of a conversation. Essentially, interaction is "hanging out." Transactions may occur when one is "hanging out," but usually they are secondary. In some interactions, head nods, facial expressions, and an occasional "uh huh" suffice. And, typically, interactions are fueled more by opinion than by fact. Doug was long on head nods and facial expressions, but his apraxia of phonation limited his "uh huhs."

Using the same tools he had available to interact—gesture, writing, drawing, and assorted media, we practiced interacting during a part of each treatment session. Our typical topics were a shared interest in vintage war movies, alternatives to Doug's 1956 BelAire, and anything he introduced in response to my "What's up?" Our time together was supplemented with Doug joining our weekly aphasia group session and interactions with other therapists, nurses, physicians, and wardmates.

C. Obtaining Speech

If we could achieve reliable phonation, I planned to attack Doug's suspected apraxia of speech. His adequate auditory comprehension and reading abilities suggested either modality would be appropriate for stimulus presentation. And, I suspected traditional motor speech drill and repetition would be most effective in restoring articulation. If it failed, we would fall back on describing how sounds were produced—"to make a /p/, you put your lips together, build up some air, and pop them"—and, if necessary, deriving sounds by modifying those he could produce into the desired target. Specific stimuli for practice would be selected from sounds Doug could produce with at least 50% accuracy in some position—initial, medial, final—in a word.

Attempts to mend Doug's apraxia of speech would await the arrival of successful, volitional phonation. And, perhaps, success with the stimuli planned for achieving phonation—vowels—would give us a head start on rolling back the apraxia of speech.

VII. TREATMENT RESULTS

A. Apraxia of Phonation

1. Methods

a. **Failure.** Some methods that have always worked do not always work. My quick fix for Doug's apraxia of phonation—a sharp push on his abdominal area while he slowly exhaled—resulted in nothing more than giving him a sore stomach. After approximately 30 trials in three successive sessions, Doug and I agreed that if at first we did not succeed, it was time to try something else.

b. **Laying on the Hands.** My backup treatment had been described by Rosenbek (1985). It involved placing my hands on Doug's thyroid cartilage during his attempts to phonate and giving him firm manual stimulation—massage, pressure, and movement of the cartilage—with simultaneous verbal coaching—"give me an /a/"—and feedback—"That's it! Hear it?"

2. The Data. Initial success—intermittent phonation during manipulation—prompted us to continue. Three vowels—/a/, /i/, and /o/—were placed in the multiple baseline design as shown in

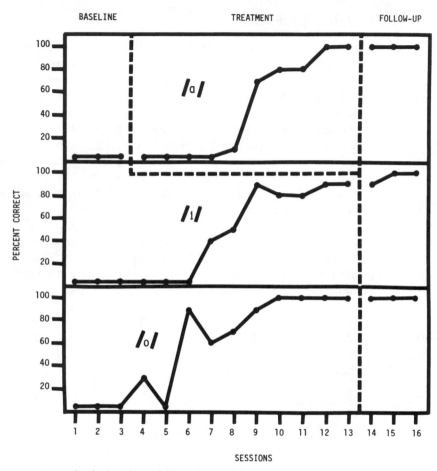

Figure 2–4. Multiple baseline design showing response to treatment for apraxia of phonation.

Figure 2–4. During sessions 1 through 3, pretreatment baseline, I requested Doug to produce each vowel 10 times, for example, "Say /a/." A correct response was clearly audible phonation of the requested vowel. Anything less—a breathy production or a phoneme other than the requested vowel—was considered incorrect. Figure 2–4 shows 0% correct for each targeted vowel in the baseline.

In sessions 4 through 13, I applied manual and verbal stimulation, 50 trials in each session, as treatment for /a/. After completing the 50 treatment trials for /a/, I conducted a daily criterion run—10

trials for each vowel as in the baseline condition, "Say _____,"
with no manual or verbal stimulation. Treatment and the criterion
run used 20 to 30 minutes of our 1-hour session.

Figure 2–4 shows Doug's phonation kicked in—30% success on
untreated /o/—in session 4. In session 6, Doug produced phonation
in 9 of 10 attempts on /o/. /i/ joined the hunt in session 7, and treated
/a/ started to get the message in session 8. By session 13, Doug was
producing acceptable phonation of each targeted vowel. In session
14, the 50 treatment trials each day were withdrawn, and performance was followed without treatment through session 16. As indicated in Figure 2–4, Doug maintained his volitional phonation at
90% to 100% accuracy for each vowel.

A multiple baseline design is used to test the efficacy of a treatment.
If performance improves more on the treated behavior than on the
untreated behaviors, one may infer a treatment effect. Doug's data
show earlier improvement on the untreated vowels—/o/ and /i/—
than on the treated vowel—/a/. Thus, the efficacy of my treatment
was not demonstrated. Few errors resulted from producing the
wrong vowel. Almost all errors were failure to phonate. For Doug,
/o/ may have been easier or my coclinicians—time and spontaneous
recovery—may have worked their magic differentially across targets. That's okay. What's bad for the design is acceptable if it is
good for the patient.

B. Communication

Simultaneous with my attempts to obtain phonation, I spent at least half
of each treatment session on functional communication. This continued
from session 1 until our time together ended. The methods were those
described earlier—employing all means at Doug's disposal to transact
and interact. When phonation arrived around session 10, it was added to
the existing armamentarium—gesture, facial expression, writing, drawing, and use of assorted media.

1. **The Methods.** As indicated earlier, we began with specific information Doug elected to transact—biography, needs, wants, and so
   on. This included a readily available orientation list—date, location, and condition—Doug used to point to in response to the inev-
   itable questions during daily, neurology bed rounds. Doug's sense
   of humor exceeded that developed during residency training and
   extended to his ability to point to each letter in "WORLD"
   backwards.

Our list of information to be transacted was kept open, and it grew to meet Doug's changing needs. Similarly, our corpus of interactive stimuli was dynamic. Doug's homework was using what we practiced in therapy in life—other treatments, the weekly aphasia group, and "bull sessions" with wardmates. My homework was gathering empirical evidence to resolve disagreement—Wallace Beery was in "Pride of the Marines," not William Bendix.

After two weeks of treatment, we put the transactional information into a PACE (Davis & Wilcox, 1985) format—Doug conveyed and I received, followed by my conveying and Doug receiving. After 3 weeks of treatment, a variety of speech-language pathology graduate students joined our sessions and were instructed to "converse" with Doug. We supplemented these conversations with prompting Doug to request information from his conversational partners. A question card—WHO, WHAT, WHEN, WHERE, WHY, and HOW—assisted Doug in putting his question train on the right track, and he followed pointing to the appropriate type of question by using gesture, writing, drawing, and media to extend and complete his question. During these conversations with students, Doug demonstrated he was a good teacher and a very patient one.

2. **The Data.** None exist. Unfortunately, I collected no data on Doug's progress during communication treatment. I could have, should have, but did not. Functional communication and its response to treatment can be quantified and qualified. No longer, usually, do I make this error of omission. With Doug, I did. And, the data are limited to pre- and posttreatment comparison on my outcome measures, particularly the CADL.

C. Apraxia of Speech

After consistent, volitional phonation was obtained—about the 3rd week of treatment—Doug demonstrated what I had expected. His speech was severely apraxic. So, I used the treatment time previously dedicated to obtaining phonation in an attempt to obtain reliable articulation.

1. **The Methods.** A phonetic inventory indicated Doug had mastered the vowels used to obtain phonation and most of the other vowels were produced correctly. For consonants, he was most successful in producing /m/ in the initial position. All other consonants were variable, and none was very robust in the initial position. But, he was usually successful with /p/ and /t/ in the final position in consonant-vowel-consonant (CVC) constructions. Therefore, I con-

structed a multiple baseline design to achieve some control of /m/, /p/, and /t/ in CVC words, for example, "mom," "meat," "mit." A PICA scoring system was employed—6 = error, 10 = self-correction, 14 = immediate, correct, but distorted. Each target sound was baselined, pretreatment. The initial treatment target was /m/, and /p/ and /t/ were followed in an untreated baseline condition. Treated, CVC /m/ stimuli were drilled for 15 minutes in each session, and data points resulted from a daily criterion run at the end of each session in which 10 CVC stimuli for each target sound were presented as in the baseline condition.

The treatment was imitative drill—"I'll say it and you say it after me. Say _____." Correct productions were confirmed by Doug and me. Incorrect productions were indicated and a repetition was presented—"No! Listen! Say _____." If the error persisted, additional help was provided—"No! Listen! Watch me! Say _____." Continuing errors led to a description of how the sound was produced and use of my hands to assist Doug in molding the desired articulatory position.

2. **The Data.** Figure 2–5 indicates baseline performance for /m/ stimuli was better than for /p/ and /t/ stimuli. Treatment of /m/ CVCs in sessions 4 through 8 showed improved performance, but there was minimal change in /p/ or /t/ CVCs. In session 9, I divided the treatment time between /m/ and /p/, with /t/ remaining in an untreated baseline. Five sessions of treating /p/ CVCs resulted in improvement. Continued treatment of /m/ CVCs showed continued good performance. Untreated /t/ CVCs did not budge.

The data in Figure 2–5 imply a treatment effect. Treated sounds, /m/ and /p/, did not improve until treated. The untreated sound, /t/, did not improve. When treatment was withdrawn, improved performance on /m/ and /p/ continued, and /t/ remained essentially unchanged.

D. Outcome

1. **A Patient's Right.** Treatment ended before I thought it would. The progress Doug made in our 2 months together prompted me to urge continued treatment. I was more excited about Doug's progress than he was, and he was more satisfied with his progress than I was. About halfway through our 2nd month, Doug indicated he was ready to go home. He had passed a driving test, qualified for dis-

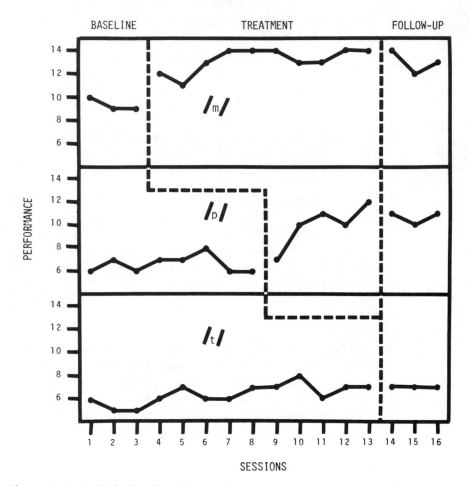

Figure 2–5. Multiple baseline design showing response to treatment for apraxia of speech.

ability income, and achieved sufficient communicative ability for his purposes. His plan was to become a person rather than a patient. That was his right, and he exercised it.

2. **Change.** Table 2–2 shows a comparison of pre- and posttreatment performance on the outcome measures. The PICA was administered 3 times—pre-, after 1 month, and after 2 months of treatment. All other measures were administered pretreatment and after 2 months of treatment.

Table 2 2. Performance on appraisal measures pre-, 3 weeks postonset, and posttreatment, 3 months postonset

Measure	Pre	Post	Difference
PICA			
Overall	33rd %ile	53rd %ile	+ 20
Gestural	54th %ile	70th %ile	+ 16
Verbal	18th %ile	26th %ile	+ 8
Graphic	35th %ile	73rd %ile	+ 38
WAB AQ	16.60	28.00	+ 11.40
Token Test Total Score	112	120	+ 8
CADL Total Score	62	113	+ 51
Apraxia of Speech Rating	7	5	− 2*

*Negative value indicates improvement

Table 2–2 and Figure 2–6 show Doug's PICA overall performance improved from the 33rd percentile at 1 month postonset, pretreatment to the 45th percentile at 2 months postonset, after 1 month of treatment; to the 53rd percentile at 3 months postonset, after 2 months of treatment. PICA gestural and graphic percentiles showed similar gains, and the verbal percentile, although lagging, also indicated improvement. Using the PICA HOAP slope method at 1 month postonset, I had predicted Doug's 33rd percentile overall performance would improve to the 43rd percentile at 3 months postonset. His performance at 3 months postonset, 53rd percentile, exceeded my prediction.

Doug's WAB AQ (Table 2–2) improved from 16.60, pretreatment, to 28.00, posttreatment. I suspect improvement on the WAB AQ was limited because of the inordinate number of speaking tasks in this measure. Four of the 5 sections in the WAB AQ—information content, fluency, repetition, and naming—require a verbal response: Doug's most impoverished communicative behavior.

The other outcome measures also showed change from pre- to posttreatment. Table 2–2 indicates Doug's *Token Test* total score improved from 112 to 120, CADL total score improved from 62 to 113, and apraxia of speech severity rating lessened from "7" to "5."

Performance on the outcome measures indicate exactly that, outcome. Several variables were at work during treatment—spontaneous recovery, treatment, and other uncontrolled influences. Thus,

Porch Index of Communicative Ability

MODALITY RESPONSE SUMMARY

Name _____D.M._____ Case No._____

Age __37__ Birthdate _7/3/46_ Sex __M__ Race_Cau.____ Handedness_Right_ ⓛ Used

Diagnosis ___Left Hemisphere CVA_____ Onset __7/30/83_____

▬▬ Date __8/22/83___ Overall __9.21_ Gestural _13.05_ Verbal __5.00_ Graphic _6.90_

∎∎∎∎∎∎∎ Date __9/30/83___ Overall _10.42_ Gestural _13.44_ Verbal __5.05_ Graphic _9.98_

∎▬∎▬∎ Date _10/28/83__ Overall __11.13_ Gestural _13.76_ Verbal __6.32_ Graphic_10.85_

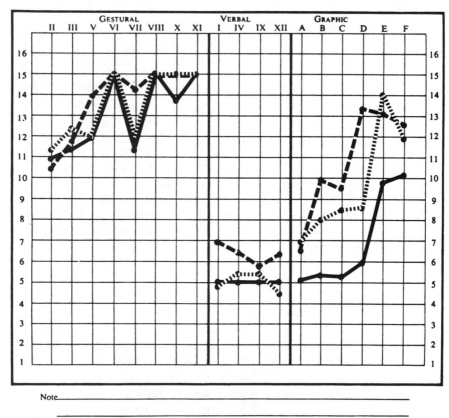

Note_____

Published by
CONSULTING PSYCHOLOGISTS PRESS
577 College Avenue   Palo Alto, California

Figure 2–6. PICA modality response summary showing change in performance from pretreatment, 3 weeks postonset, to posttreatment, 3 months postonset.

although I cannot attribute Doug's improvement to the treatment provided (efficacy); I can demonstrate he improved (outcome).

E. Follow Up

Approximately 1 month after Doug terminated treatment, he returned for a follow-up neurology and speech pathology appointment. Time permitted administration of the PICA and a brief conversation about how he was doing.

Figure 2–7 indicates Doug's overall PICA percentile had slid slightly from the 53rd at the end of treatment to the 51st 1 month later. I considered the 2-percentile dip was not cause for alarm. Doug agreed. He conveyed life at home was "good," and he filled his day with television, tinkering with his car, and household chores assigned by his mother. He had re-entered his social circle, and his evenings and weekends consisted of "hanging out with the guys." He had no plans for work, and he definitely had no plans for continuing treatment. I wished him well and indicated treatment's door remained open. He thanked me and conveyed he would let me know. He hasn't.

VIII. DISCUSSION

A. Retrospection

Doug's management probably falls under that broad, ill-defined adjective called "traditional." I did nothing innovative, new, or different from what most clinicians, I suspect, would have done. Doug's communicative deficits were "mixed"—aphasia, apraxia of speech, and apraxia of phonation. They were attacked separately but simultaneously. I believed he needed consistent, reliable phonation before speech would be within reach, so I went after that first. However, during the time we awaited the onset of phonation, I believed he needed a means to communicate. So, we developed that simultaneously with our work on phonation. He succeeded in achieving both. Once he could produce reliable phonation, we attempted to add some control over his articulatory gestures by working on his apraxia of speech. Our success with achieving voice and functional communication was greater than our success in achieving speech. I believe, with additional time, we could have rolled back more of Doug's apraxia of speech. But, I do not know.

B. Realism

Doug received 2 months of treatment—once a day, five days a week—for a total of approximately 40 sessions. This is not an unrealistic inten-

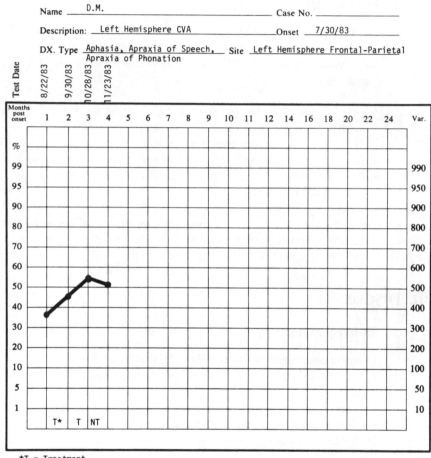

Porch **I**ndex of **C**ommunicative **A**bility

APHASIA RECOVERY CURVE

Name ____D.M._____ Case No. _____

Description: ___Left Hemisphere CVA_____ Onset ___7/30/83_____

DX. Type _Aphasia, Apraxia of Speech,_ Site _Left Hemisphere Frontal-Parietal_
          Apraxia of Phonation

.*T = Treatment
NT = No Treatment

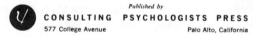

Published by
CONSULTING PSYCHOLOGISTS PRESS
577 College Avenue   Palo Alto, California

Figure 2–7. PICA aphasia recovery curve showing change from pretreatment, 3 weeks postonset, to follow up, 4 months postonset.

sity and duration of treatment, even by today's standards of shrinking services. Doug and I believed the treatment helped, but we do not know. The outcome was good. He improved. The efficacy is unknown. Together, we negotiated treatment's content. I recommended, and Doug decided. Alone, he specified treatment's end. During our last visit, Doug conveyed he was doing "okay." Some impairment and disability persisted. His handicap, I suspect, was more than he would have elected, but the amount that persisted seemed tolerable to him. Doug demonstrates that aphasic people, including those who have coexisting apraxia of phonation and apraxia of speech, improve. They do not recover. The amount of acceptable improvement will differ among patients and between patient and clinician. Doug was willing to accept less than I was. Good for him.

IX. REFERENCES

Albert, M., Sparks, R., & Helm, N. (1973). Melodic intonation therapy for aphasia. *Archives of Neurology, 29,* 130–131.

Bowman, C. A., Hodson, B. W., & Simpson, R. K. (1980). Oral apraxia and aphasic misarticulations. In R. H. Brookshire (Ed.), *Clinical aphasiology: Conference proceedings* (pp. 89–95). Minneapolis: BRK Publishers.

Butfield, E. (1958). Rehabilitation of the dysphasic patient. *Speech Pathology Therapy, 1,* 9–17, 60–65.

Darley, F. L. (1982). *Aphasia.* Philadelphia: W. B. Saunders.

Davis, G. A., & Wilcox, M. J. (1985). *Adult aphasia rehabilitation: Applied pragmatics.* San Diego: College-Hill Press.

DeRenzi, E., Pieczuro, A., & Vignolo, L. A. (1966). Oral apraxia and aphasia. *Cortex, 2,* 50–73.

Duffy, J. R. (1995). *Motor speech disorders: Substrates, differential diagnosis, and management.* St. Louis: Mosby.

Dworkin, J. P., & Abkarian, G. G. (1996). Treatment of phonation in a patient with apraxia and dysarthria secondary to severe closed head injury. *Journal of Medical Speech-Language Pathology, 4,* 105–115.

Goodglass, H., & Kaplan, E. (1983). *Boston Diagnostic Aphasia Examination.* Philadelphia: Lea & Febiger.

Holland, A. L. (1980). *Communicative Abilities in Daily Living.* Baltimore: University Park Press.

Kertesz, A. (1982). *Western Aphasia Battery.* New York: Grune & Stratton.

LaPointe, L. L., & Wertz, R. T. (1974). Oral-movement abilities and articulatory characteristics of brain-injured adults. *Perceptual and Motor Skills, 39,* 39–46.

Lebrun, Y. (1990). *Mutism.* London: Whurr Publishers Ltd.

Martin, A. D. (1974). Some objections to the term apraxia of speech. *Journal of Speech and Hearing Disorders, 39,* 53–64.

Mohr, J. P. (1980). Revision of Broca aphasia and the syndrome of Broca's area infarction and its implications in aphasia theory. In R. H. Brookshire (Ed.), *Clinical aphasiology: Conference proceedings* (pp. 1–16). Minneapolis: BRK Publishers.

Porch, B. E. (1967). *The Porch Index of Communicative Ability.* Palo Alto, CA: Consulting Psychologists Press.

Rosenbek, J. C. (1985). Treating apraxia of speech. In D. F. Johns (Ed.), *Clinical management of neurogenic communicative disorders* (2nd ed., pp. 267–312). Boston: Little, Brown.

Rosenbek, J. C., LaPointe, L. L., & Wertz, R. T. (1989). *Aphasia: A clinical approach.* Austin, TX: PRO-ED.

Simpson, M. B., & Clark, A. R. (1989). Clinical management of apractic mutism. In P. Square-Storer (Ed.), *Acquired apraxia of speech in aphasic adults* (pp. 241–266). London: Taylor & Francis.

Spreen, O., & Benton, A. L. (1969). *Neurosensory center comprehensive examination for aphasia* (rev. ed.). Victoria, BC: University of Victoria.

Square-Storer, P. (Ed.). (1989). *Acquired apraxia of speech in aphasic adults.* London: Taylor & Francis.

Vignolo, L. A. (1964). Evolution of aphasia and language rehabilitation: A retrospective study. *Cortex, 1,* 344–367.

Webb, W. G., & Love, R. J. (1974, November). *The efficacy of cuing techniques with apraxic-aphasics.* Paper presented to the American Speech and Hearing Association, Las Vegas, NV.

Wertz, R. T. (1984). Response to treatment in patients with apraxia of speech. In J. C. Rosenbek, M. R. McNeil, & A. E. Aronson (Eds.), *Apraxia of speech: Physiology, acoustics, linguistics, management* (pp. 257–276). San Diego: College-Hill Press.

Wertz, R. T., LaPointe, L. L., & Rosenbek, J. C. (1984). *Apraxia of speech in adults.* San Diego: Singular Publishing Group.

CHAPTER

3

A Strategy for Improving Oral Naming in an Individual With a Phonological Access Impairment

AUDREY L. HOLLAND, Ph.D.

I. BACKGROUND

A. Phonological Access Impairments

1. **Definition.** As used here, "phonological access impairment" is a cluster of problems that includes a prominent dissociation of oral and written single word production in aphasia. This dissociation can be fruitfully examined from the perspective of Patterson and

Shewall's processing model (1987). Most models suggest that phonological processing is a requirement for writing. The Patterson and Shewall model (1987) does not. Rather, it examines the transduction of spoken and written words from recognition to comprehension and production in such a way as to permit independent access from the cognitive system (semantics) to phonological and orthographic output lexicons. Figure 3–1 shows relevant portions of the Patterson and Shewall model, with the area hypothesized to produce the oral/written word dissociation shaded in gray.

2. **Historical perspective.** Over the past decade or so, there has been a growing interest in the study of brain-damaged individuals who have selective impairments or surprising dissociations of language functions. Some examples involving spoken words include individuals who have difficulty naming pictures of specific classes of nouns, such as fruits and vegetables (Farah & Wallace, 1992), or inanimate as opposed to living things and foods (Warrington & Shallice, 1984), or who have difficulty naming verbs but not nouns or vice versa (Caramazza & Hillis, 1991; Zingeser & Berndt, 1988). Such patients have been intensively studied largely because their patterns of skills and deficits are useful for shedding light on how the brain processes language.

One particularly interesting dissociation involves individuals whose written output is substantially better than their speech. Shelton and Weinrich (in press) report that at least eight individuals with such dissociations have been described. (Assal, Buttet, & Jolivet, 1981; Bub & Kertesz, 1982; Caramazza, Berndt, & Basili, 1983; Ellis, Miller, & Sin, 1983; Hier & Mohr, 1977; Kremin, 1987; Levine, Calvanio, & Popovics, 1982; Patterson & Shewall, 1987; Shelton & Weinrich, in press). Most of these patients have been extensively studied and their performances compared on a variety of written and spoken tasks related to cognitive neuropsychological processing models. As Shelton and Weinrich (in press) point out, these patients directly challenge longstanding beliefs that the ability to write (at least in individuals who are not deaf) depends on the ability first to generate an internal phonological representation and then to translate that representation into the appropriate graphemes. If it can be demonstrated that, following brain damage, access to written forms remains intact in some individuals who have at best limited access to their spoken equivalents, then there is not an inviolable link between written and spoken routes and the underlying semantic system.

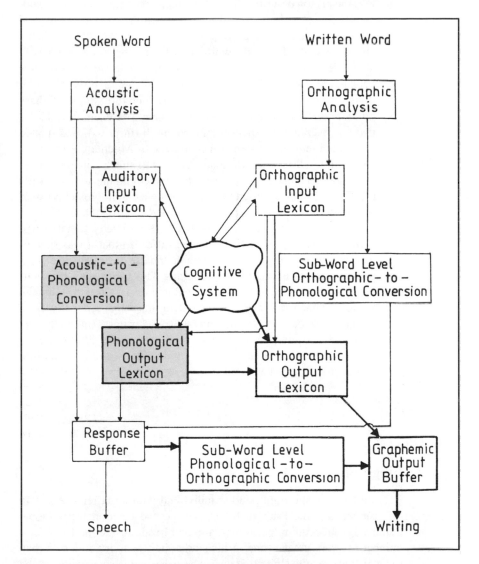

Figure 3–1. Patterson and Shewall's model for recognition, comprehension, and production of single words. (From "Speak and Spell: Dissociations and Word Class Effects" by K. Patterson and C. Shewell, p. 274, in *The Cognitive Neuropsychology of Language,* edited by M. Coltheant, G. G. Satori, and R. Job, 1987. London: LEA, Ltd. Copyright 1987. Reprinted by permission of Erlbaum (UK) Taylor & Francis, Hove, UK.)

RR, the person described here, has excellent comprehension of spoken discourse and intact, if slow, silent reading. He has severe oral anomia, but no motor speech impairments. He also has a remarkable ability to write the single words that he can neither say nor read aloud. RR's dissociated oral and written single-word skills have been extensively evaluated (in preparation), as have the dissociations of similar subjects reported in the literature. Some of these other individuals have undergone treatment. For example, AE, the patient described by Shelton and Weinrich (in press), was treated for written sentence production conducted by Mitchum, Haendiges, and Berndt (1993). AE was also a subject in an experimental treatment approach using computerized visual communication (C-VIC) (1997), and an unspecified treatment designed to improve his use of past tense morphology, a problem that RR does not have. None of the similar patients received treatment that directly targeted oral word retrieval. Thus, RR's treatment differs in that it was specifically designed to develop and promote the use of strategies to compensate for his phonological difficulties. This treatment is the focus of this report. The question of clinical interest is: Once the clinician has determined that a given patient profits only minimally from phonological cueing, cannot generate sound patterns internally, and cannot consistently read words aloud after successfully writing them, what can be done to help the individual with his or her oral word-retrieval problem?

II. THE PATIENT

A. Biography

RR is a 68-year-old, right-handed individual with a master's degree in international affairs. Prior to his stroke, he had been an international publishing and printing consultant and had lived outside the USA for a number of years. At the time of his stroke, he was living in a suburban town in the eastern United States, where he was also serving as the mayor. In addition to his native English, RR spoke Portuguese and Spanish fluently before his stroke. Since the stroke, however, RR reports being much more aphasic in Portuguese than in English, and he has avoided trying to speak Spanish. He further noted that trying to communicate with his monolingual Portuguese-speaking friends also hampered his English for a day or so subsequently. RR is married, and has one grown son. He has wide interests, ranging from politics to music and history. He has always been an avid reader and an accomplished (published) writer and correspondent.

B. Medical History

Hospital records indicated that in January 1991, RR suffered a middle cerebral artery occlusion. No further details concerning localization of the lesion at that time appear in the records. However, a volumetric CT scan, done at the University of Iowa Department of Radiology in February 1995 revealed a very large left hemisphere lesion, with virtual destruction of Brodmann's areas 22, 39, and 40. (See Figure 3–2 for a volumetric reconstruction of his left and right hemispheres.) Within 1 day of his stroke, RR attempted to communicate by drawing rudimentary maps and writing single words. RR has no residual motor impairments, although he complains of considerably constrained vocal range and "tightness" in his larynx when he talks. Comparison of his present speaking voice with a videotape made before the stroke confirms this voice change.

C. Language Description

The most striking initial impression of RR was how easily he wrote the words that he could not say. He was a skilled communicator, although he overused a limited number of words. (For example, good things were typically either described as "interesting" or "terrific," depending on his degree of enthusiasm; bad things were "terrible.") When he could not say the substantive word he was searching for, he correctly and effortlessly wrote it on a small pad of paper he always carried, then trusted his listeners to be able to read it (even upside down), and continued to talk. He used this strategy to discuss a very wide range of topics. Possibly because of the category's arbitrary nature, proper names presented particular difficulty for RR. Paraphasias (semantic and phonemic) almost never occurred. He spoke extremely slowly, and his speech contained many false starts, revisions, and pauses, perhaps in an effort to avoid making a paraphasic error. Misspellings were relatively rare; paragraphias were few and likely to be intrusions of correctly spelled Portuguese words. RR was largely unable to say or read aloud the single words he wrote. He could not (and still cannot) write spontaneous phrases or sentences. RR reports that his ability to read was "almost as good as before, but slow." Thus, this puzzling man could write single words, speak in labored sentences, read novels, follow normal conversation—but could not do the more basic tasks on which such skills presumably depend.

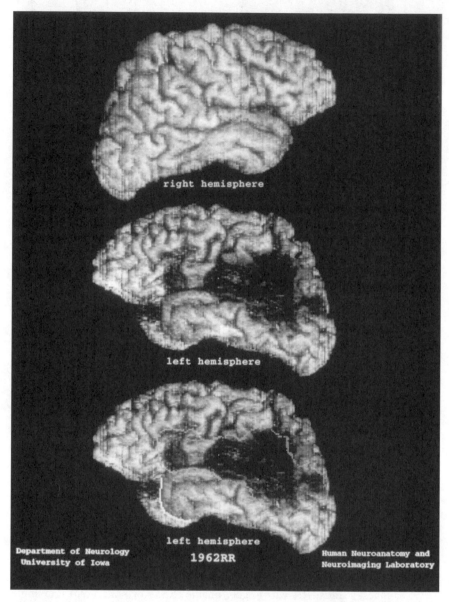

Figure 3–2. Volumetric reconstruction of RR's left and right hemispheres.

Following is a transcription of a 5-minute sample of RR's speech. He is beginning to describe the book he has just completed, *The First Man* by Albert Camus.[1]

Well, I just recently. . . . The First Man of uh, of uh (wrote Camus). I liked him very much years ago and uh, recently——It had come out recently here and uh, I bought it. I hadn't realized———I knew he was uh from uh—he was a uh Frenchman, but he was, he was he was from (wrote Algiers). And uh, it was interesting. First of all, uh, his mother was———they were really from Spain originally. The father was from France but had been living there (pointed to the word Algiers) and he had been an, he had been, he had been, the father had been (wrote ophanage)—the father had been an orphan. The mother was (wrote laundress). They had various children, but from the mother—the father—(wrote grandmother) lived there and the father, the father and because———Wait a minute. Let me go back and tell you what happened.

The father and the mother they had a boy 'fore him (Q? A brother for Albert?) Yes. Just before he was in the (wrote war). Number 1. They were—and he was born and almost immediately the father had to go to France and was killed. (Q? So that left the mother and the grandmother?) Yes. Exactly. They were extremely poor. So much that at one point he mentioned that they, they never had, never had a (wrote book). They did not even have a (wrote newspaper). They had nothing. Nothing. They did not use (wrote electricity). When things were———at night they finally would put a light (wrote kerosene).

D. Previous Management

Following his stroke, RR consistently sought and sporadically received individual and group speech-language therapy in his local area for 3 years. Detailed summaries are unavailable, but it was reported that he made "considerable progress" in treatment. RR reports that the discrepancy between spoken and written word retrieval has been a prominent and consistent characteristic of his poststroke language. In previous therapy, RR was introduced to unspecified computer activities "and had begun to develop some limited word processing skills." He also worked on writing dictated words and sentences.

A significant feature of his management was that he was highly motivated and followed self-organized speaking practice regimens as consistently as others might undertake daily physical exercise. RR reports generating written word lists, which he repeatedly practiced reading

[1]RR's written words are preserved in the transcript and indicated by underlining.

aloud. He also reports setting aside a few hours each day for silent reading.

RR actively advocates for other aphasic individuals to develop and participate in aphasia groups and believes strongly that aphasic individuals should take an active and responsible role in managing their own difficulties. He organized and began leading his first self-help aphasia group in 1991.

RR moved to Arizona in 1994 and was referred to our clinic by his previous therapist. He has been driving 2 hours to our clinic each week for individual and group therapy since September 1994, paying for his treatment out of pocket or by serving as a paid research subject. At the time of this report, RR had founded three aphasia groups in his local community.

III. LANGUAGE APPRAISAL

A. Rationale and Methods

A general inventory of aphasia, as well as a number of other measures designed to provide information on the characteristics and the extent of RR's processing difficulties were used.

1. **Basic Aphasia Test.** First, in an effort to develop a consistent data base for our aphasia clinic, we use the *Western Aphasia Battery* (WAB, Kertesz, 1982), often supplemented with the *Aphasia Diagnostic Profile* (ADP, Helm-Estabrooks, 1992). The WAB was administered to RR.

2. **Additional measures.** Governing the choice of additional appraisal material was the need to gain information about RR's unusual pattern of communication problems, which were not readily explainable from the inventory approach of a basic aphasia test.

   I wanted to understand RR's problems as fully as I could by reading about similar cases and using testing material that others had found useful, supplemented by some other tasks that I thought might provide additional information. I felt there were two issues: (1) The extent of this speaking/writing dissociation of naming and its underlying processing deficit. (2) The necessity for knowing more about the problem to provide effective treatment. Measures for each of these aspects are described briefly:

a. **Extent of dissociation.** For this, oral and written naming performance was measured using well controlled confrontation naming tasks developed by Berndt and her associates. One set consisted of 140 pictures (7 blocks of 20 pictures each) developed by Raymer and Berndt (1996) to assess frequency and regularity effects on word retrieval. The second set compared noun and verb naming of stimuli with equivalent frequencies (Berndt, Mitchum, Haendiges, & Sandson, 1997).

b. **Underlying processing deficit.** RR's ability to manipulate acoustic codes internally was tested using the following measures (or parts of them) from the *Psycholinguistic Assessments of Language Processing in Aphasia* (PALPA, Kay, Lesser, & Coltheart, 1992). These measures were chosen because they represented processing skills tested by other investigators whose patients seemed most closely to resemble RR.

(1) Single-word repetition tasks (high and low frequency, high and low imageability).
(2) Writing real and pseudowords to dictation.
(3) Rhyming judgment tasks, which were presented orally and in writing.
(4) Written lexical decision tasks in which RR was asked which of a corpus of real words and phonologically plausible nonwords were words and which were not.

B. Results

1. **WAB.** RR achieved an aphasia quotient (AQ) of 60.2, on his first WAB, given in June 1994. His overall pattern of language assets and deficits was consistent with classification of conduction aphasia. His poorest performances were in repetition and naming, particularly confrontation naming and category fluency. An unexpected finding was that RR had some difficulty with single-word comprehension, despite his otherwise good performance on the test's linguistically more complex (and contextual) comprehension tasks. (It should be noted that as a result of his continuing involvement with our aphasia clinic, RR receives a yearly WAB. The second WAB was completed in 1995. His AQ at that time was calculated as 62.8 and is the basis for comparisons made later in this paper.)

Although the WAB classified his disorder as conduction aphasia, it should be noted that RR's speech output was atypical for that syndrome in that, although he was largely fluent, his speech lacked phonemic paraphasias and *conduites d'approche*. Rather, when RR was permitted to respond only verbally, his error responses were either statements such as "I can't do it," or "Nope," or long silences that were marked by nonverbal oral movements that are difficult to describe but did not seem apracticlike in nature.

2. Additional Measures

a. **Dissociation extent.** The following confrontation naming measures all involved comparisons between RR's written and spoken ability to access the lexicon.

(1) **Raymer and Berndt pictures.** 140 pictures controlled for frequency and regularity (1996). RR's spoken and written performances were strikingly different. On oral tasks, he correctly named 25 of the total set, while he correctly wrote (and mostly correctly spelled) 127. (This was not a practice effect. For each block, its order of presentation in the two modalities was randomly determined and presentation was separated by a week.) Performance within each block of 20 pictures was remarkably stable. Typically RR named 3 or 4 correctly, and wrote 18–20 of the names correctly. No frequency or regularity effects were noted.

(2) **Noun-verb naming tasks matched for frequency** (Berndt, et al., 1997). Eight of 30 nouns, and 5 of 30 verbs were correctly named orally, with 29 nouns and 25 verbs, respectively, correctly written. Thus, the difference between spoken and written performance continued to be striking and neither frequency nor part-of-speech effects were evident.

b. **Processing tasks.** These tasks provide ways to understand how RR manipulated acoustic codes.

(1) **Single-word repetition tasks** (high and low frequency, high and low imageability). Only the low-imagery, low-frequency words presented significant repetition difficulty (10/20 correct). All words tested were within RR's repetition span, determined by WAB to be three syllables, independent of whether the stimulus was a long word such as "information" or a short sentence of the same number of syllables, such as "Buy a new coat."

(2) **Writing real and pseudowords to dictation.** RR performed badly (8 of 20) writing real words to dictation, and was unable to write pseudowords at all (0/30).

(3) **Rhyming judgment tasks.** RR's performance on both listening and reading rhyming tasks was no better than chance (17/30).

(4) **Written lexical decision task.** RR's performance was perfect (40/40).

V. DIAGNOSIS

A. Patterns of Strengths and Weaknesses

I believe that the basis for treatment of an aphasic individual requires a comparison of strengths and weaknesses. It is insufficient to diagnose a patient merely by type and severity of aphasia. RR's case is an excellent example of the problems inherent in a diagnosis such as "moderately-severe conduction aphasia" gleaned from his WAB scores. The attempt to pinpoint the extent and nature of his dissociation confirmed his strengths and weaknesses, as listed in Table 3–1, and provided leads for making clinical decisions and focusing RR's treatment.

1. **Considerations.** The results presented in Table 3–1 suggest that RR's problems are primarily phonological. More specifically, phonological access difficulties are at the root of his dissociated oral and written naming. The notion that he has only a phonological access impairment also would help to explain RR's unusual ability to do quite complex linguistic tasks—sophisticated comprehension of conversation, plays, novels, and nonfiction—with relative ease in the face of severe impairments on simple phonological tasks. (For example, using his writing strategy to supplement his speech, RR can discuss a novel he is reading, but he cannot recite the alphabet.) All of the PALPA tasks and most of the WAB tasks on which he performed poorly were devoid of context (linguistic and otherwise) and, therefore, required RR to rely only on phonological aspects of the stimuli he heard. When RR is reading connected discourse or involved in conversation, he is receiving multiple contextual cues to help him. Among these are probability effects related to syntax, linguistic redundancy, and (in speech at least) prosodic features. He is able to take advantage of all these features that are missing from single-word tasks. How does this type of information help to explain his speech production and oral naming problems? RR

Table 3–1. RR's language strengths and weaknesses revealed by assessment and observation/interaction.

Strengths/Weaknesses	Source of Evidence	Effects
Strengths		
Excellent comprehension (discourse and text reading)	WAB, conversational skills, ability to read newspapers, fiction, nonfiction	Context enhances performances
Spontaneous single-word writing	WAB, Berndt et al. (1997) tests, conversation	Semantic system largely intact
Lexical decision	PALPA subtest	Semantic orthographic system largely intact
Weaknesses		
Cannot reliably access semantics from minimal acoustic cues	WAB, observation	Questionable single-word comprehension skills
Poor phonological memory	WAB, PALPA repetition tasks	Acoustic to phonological conversion fails when span (3 syllables) is exceeded.
Poor grapheme-to-phoneme conversion	WAB, conversation	Cannot write pseudowords to dictation, minimal ability with real words written while talking
Minimal internal sound patterns?	PALPA	Chance performance with rhymes

demonstrates his intact semantic system when he writes the word he searches for. But once the word is written, the phonological deficit reemerges, and he faces the same difficulties in phonological interpretation that block his abilities to write the words that others say to him. RR, himself, describes his problem most succinctly. As he was attempting, most painfully, to perform the rhyming tasks, he noted, "I have no sound patterns for these in my head."[2]

---

[2]In retrospect, I probably could have saved us both a great deal of time and effort if I had simply believed RR.

V. PROGNOSIS

A. Prognostic Signs

Few of us seriously believe that we treat the *disorder* of aphasia. Rather, the individual who has the disorder is central to our work. Linguistic aspects of the aphasia are important, to be sure, but they must be placed in the context of the natural history of recovery and the personal characteristics of each aphasic individual. My belief is that these latter factors become more important as the time from the aphasia-producing stroke increases, that is, when we no longer can count on spontaneous recovery to aid us in our work.

1. **Signs from the natural history of aphasia.** Most of the traditional signs would suggest that RR's prognosis for further recovery was not particularly good. He was more than 3 years postonset of aphasia when he first contacted us; he appeared already to have made substantial progress as the result of spontaneous recovery, clinical intervention, and self-discipline. Although his age was not a deterrent to recovery, it was easy to question whether driving a 250-mile round trip at least once a week for therapy at our clinic might result in fatigue, hardly a favorable prognostic sign.

   The very specificity of RR's disorder was a deterrent. And so was the fact that no one, neither RR's previous clinicians, nor clinicians who had worked with the similar cases in the literature, had apparently developed or carried out a plan for managing the phonological problem. Yet to work on another problem, such as written sentence production, did not appeal to RR, who made it clear that his difficulty in saying specific words was his most frustrating and perplexing problem and the one for which he sought help.

2. **Neuropsychological and personal characteristics.** RR had been assessed with a number of neuropsychological tests and ancillary measures. Negative features included a tendency to respond too quickly, before tasks were fully explained, as well as some difficulties in changing set (as measured by the *Wisconsin Card Sorting Test*) and in allocating resources when competing stimuli were present. Among his strengths were excellent spatial organization, strong performance on the *Raven's Progressive Matrices* and on visual paired associate learning, which suggested, along with his obviously high intelligence, that he was probably capable of new learning. He was objective about his problems and made it clear that he had no unrealistic goals or illusions about how much progress he

might make. However in my view, the most important attributes contributing to a positive prognosis were his determination and motivation to work on improving his spoken language.

B. Expected Outcome

I have never been particularly concerned about time postonset as a negative prognostic sign for recovery, primarily because so much of the experimental treatment research with good results has been conducted on chronic patients. In RR's case, few factors seemed to me to outweigh the combination of his motivation and my curiosity. I did not have any expectations concerning outcome, rather I was interested in "giving it a try." I communicated as much to RR. I hoped to help RR use his writing to facilitate his oral word production.

RR was already a functional communicator, in the sense of being able to communicate basic needs and to carry out the types of transactions and interactions described by Jon Lyon in Chapter 9. Functional outcomes, therefore, had to be considered as improvements on far more elusive issues, such as improving RR's quality of life.

VI. FOCUSING THE TREATMENT

A. Rationale

Work with RR centered on developing strategies for accessing phonological information. Because writing single words was clearly his most effective strategy for word finding, writing played a major role in the attempt to make phonological access easier for RR. I did not even entertain the notion that phonological access routes could be restored by practice. Rather, the focus was on ways to *circumvent* what are probably the normal processes for accessing phonology—what RR described as "having sound patterns in his head." For RR's particular constellation of problems, if normal phonological access routes were impaired, then clinical intervention had to center on alternative mechanisms.

B. Methods

This chapter portion has two main sections. The first summarizes the extensive treatment phase designed to help RR develop bridges between orthographic and phonological information. The second section presents in detail an approach to training more systematic use of these bridges for spontaneous word generation.

1. **Bridges to phonology: The Autocue.** Early work with RR involved a modification of the phonemic self-cueing technique developed by Nickels (1992) in which "bridges," or "relays," systematically relate graphemes to phonemes. (For example, a "bridge" might be the association first of a visualized snake with the grapheme s and then with the /s/ phoneme.) Nickels calls these relays, or bridges, "autocues." Autocues are first explained, then associated, then practiced with a few words beginning with the grapheme/phoneme in training. For example, the aphasic speaker is trained, on seeing the word "sit," to associate its initial grapheme to the *initial sound* of the bridge word "snake" before attempting to say it aloud. In RR's case, using these autocues to trigger *internally visualized* words was the goal. This laborious and intellectually demanding approach to grapheme-phoneme conversion was a focus of therapy during once-weekly sessions for approximately a year-and-a-half, approximately 60 sessions. RR learned grapheme-to-phoneme autocues for most English consonants. In addition, he learned the simple strategy of opening his mouth, should the initial sound of a word be a vowel. He was successful at saying words on alphabetically arranged lists, regardless of whether they were self-generated or provided by the therapist. And his oral confrontation naming also improved considerably. At one point in this learning process, RR noted to his clinician that he could not orally name the picture "praying" because "I haven't learned the (gestured praying and wrote 'p') thing yet." However, it was extremely difficult for RR to use the autocue strategy in conversation or even in naming to definition. This was largely because initially writing, then searching for and finding the correct phoneme, and then attempting the word was very slow. Thus, the autocue competed poorly with the already effective writing strategy. Finally RR's practice with printed word lists was very different from on-line oral word retrieval in conversation and transfer to that skill was correspondingly difficult.

Lesser (1989) has pointed out that retrieval of names in natural discourse is a much more complex communicative and social activity than what she called the "metalinguistic act" of naming, as exemplified by confrontation naming or reading word lists aloud. To approach using autocues in natural discourse, RR next spent 16 sessions using autocues in relation to naming attributes of a given pictured object. This was felt to be a closer approximation to word retrieval in discourse, but still under clinician control. This phase of his treatment was an adaptation of a semantic (as opposed to phonological) self-cueing technique developed by Lowell, Beeson, and Holland (1995). The rationale was that, as RR already had good semantic access, he could be counted on to retrieve attributes, and the clinician could provide the constraints necessary for RR to stop and name the attribute after writing it. Although the approach was challenging to RR, it remained difficult to require him to use auto-cues, and, in addition, there was virtually no carryover to conversation. Therefore, the decision was made to formalize an approach for linking RR's autocue skills with his writing strategy. It is this portion of his therapy that I describe in detail.

2. **Training a strategy for using autocues in self-generated speech.** For aphasic learners to use what might initially seem to be cumbersome communicative strategies, they must understand them and become committed to using them. Thus, the decision to undertake this new phase of treatment was a joint one. The approach and its intended goal were clearly explained, and its potential value in improving his spontaneous speech was reinforced. RR was willing to try a new approach, even though it required a conscious break from his standard (and successful, if awkward) writing strategy. Incidentally, one of RR's functional goals was to use fewer of the pads of paper he kept in his shirt pocket for use on occasions when he needed to write his words, and consequently to lessen his daily contributions to the deforestation of America.

To move treatment toward self-generated speech, category naming, an even closer approximation to on-line word retrieval in discourse, was used. In confrontation naming, the therapist controls the options. In providing words that typify a category, the speaker has greater control of the options, more analogous to, but far from identical to, word finding in self-generated discourse. RR agreed to the constraint that during training, regardless of the exemplars he chose, he would not be permitted to go on to an additional exemplar before he said the one just written. The goal was to use the word-retrieval strategy in a way that did not feel awkward to RR or his listeners. We deliberately limited this treatment to 11 sessions, to bring it within the scope of current reimbursement practices. That is, if RR had arrived on our doorstep with his skills as they were at the point this treatment began, and if we had been authorized to conduct 12 sessions (including assessment), could we have demonstrated a change?

Table 3–2 lists the therapy topics for 11, 45-minute treatment sessions, conducted over 3½ months. These topics were chosen to be challenging and to provide opportunities for evoking proper names to increase RR's need to use his writing strategy. Topics for the

Table 3–2. Topics for category naming: "Think of words that are related specifically to this topic."

	Phases 1, 2, 4	Phase 3	Homework
Session 1	Medical	Religion	Wild West
Session 2	Latin America	Russia	Movie titles
Session 3	Buildings and monuments	Natural sites	World holidays
Session 4	Music	Printing/publishing	American politicians
Session 5	Renaissance	Drama and dance	Break (no homework)
Session 6	World War I	Weather	Famous animals
Session 7	Cleaning terms	Cooking	Herbs and spices
Session 8	Sports	Travel	Time and space
Session 9	Print media	Television	Insects
Session 10	Tools and utensils	Emotions	Water
Session 11	Vehicles	Body parts	Games

clinical sessions were conceptualized as pairs of related concepts and randomly designated as testing or treatment topics. The focus of the treatment sessions was *self-generation* of words for using the autocues as described previously. Each session had five phases. All responses were tape recorded for later verification and transcribed on line by the clinician (ALH) and a student clinician, with some help from Pelagie M. Beeson (2 sessions). Misspellings were basically ignored during the treatment, but they were maintained in the transcriptions.

RR also completed five practice sessions at home each week. In these sessions, he was expected to write and then attempt to say 10 words a day on an assigned topic using the "crib sheet" shown. RR was not expected to produce new words in his home practice each day, but was encouraged to mix words from a previous day with new ones, as he wished. RR recorded all his words on special forms and put a check mark beside each one correctly said. Data consisted of the number of words correctly produced. RR's self-monitoring was not considered to be an issue for this homework, primarily because his consistent self-monitoring error was rejection of correct responses. In view of this, his homework record was considered to be a conservative estimate of his performance.

The phases of this treatment and their durations were as follows:

  a. **Category naming (Phase 1: No Writing).** During this 5-minute period, the first session topic was announced and RR was asked to generate exemplars aloud. No pencil was provided. No feedback was given.

b. **Demonstration (Phase 2: Writing required).** This phase was also 5 minutes long. Using the same category, RR was given a pencil and required to write each exemplar he thought of and to say it immediately after writing it. He was reminded of his autocues, if necessary, or in some instances prompted with the initial sound. If he still could not say the word he had written, the clinician said it, and it was broken down into syllables until he could repeat it. Because the goal was to evoke a spoken response for each written word, he never moved on until a correct oral production was achieved. At the end of this phase, his performance with writing was compared to performance without writing, and the (usually) slightly higher number of spoken exemplars was explained as a function of the facilitative effects of the writing activity on speaking.

c. **Practice (Phase 3: Writing required).** Next, RR was given a 25-minute practice period in which a new topic was introduced, and the procedures of the demonstration phase were followed. In this phase, as in all phases of this treatment, RR was required to generate his own exemplars. RR was initially required to follow the sequence of writing, then saying each word before moving on to another word. However, when RR began occasionally to write and say the words simultaneously, this stringent requirement was modified. Throughout each session, the crib sheet was displayed, which included the following reminders about maximizing speech production: As with Phase 2, all words generated were recorded.

CRIB SHEET
1. Do not hold your breath.
2. Speak on exhalation.
3. Breathe out.
4. Get the first sound under control before talking.
5. Give yourself permission to:
    a. Be flexible. If you can't say the word you want, let go and think of an alternative.
    b. Relax
    c. Take a chance. Paraphasias are at least in the ballpark.

d. **Posttesting (Phase 4: Pencil provided but not required).** In the 5-minute posttest, RR returned to the untrained topic of the pretest and the demonstration. A pencil was made available, but RR was not specifically encouraged to use it. Rather, he was simply reminded that he did better at talking and writing than at talking alone and that it was generally easier and more natural for his communication partners if RR said the words, even if it was more time-consuming. The words RR produced were recorded, and it was noted if he spoke, spoke and wrote, or simply wrote the words he generated.

e. **Conversational sample (Phase 5).** Each session ended with a 5-minute conversation, each on a different current-events topic. RR and two clinicians participated. Each conversation was tape recorded, and in addition, both clinicians counted on-line the number and manner of productions of the substantive words RR generated.

For homework, RR's responses and his recorded evaluations of his accuracy were used as data. Abbreviated session and homework forms, and instructions are provided in Table 3–3.

VII. RESULTS

A. Reliability Considerations

An important consideration was to develop a brief treatment regimen that other clinicians could use. For this reason, reliability measures were chosen that could be used easily in ongoing clinical interactions. For these 11 sessions all responses and their form of production (written, written and spoken, spoken) were transcribed on line. Only responses that were agreed on by the clinician and the clinical assistant constituted the data used for computing these results. A simple data form was developed and used for each session. Because word generation under conditions of this treatment was a relatively slow process, the 100% agreement required was relatively easy to achieve for Phases 1–4. Phase 5 was problematical, however; in addition to transcribing form and content of the response, it was necessary for both participant-observers to agree if the response was a substantive word.

This approach to reliability is quite conservative, particularly for the homework sessions reported below, because of RR's tendency to underestimate his performances. However, the advantage of being simple and easy to approximate in ongoing clinical work was thought to outweigh its conservatism.

Table 3–3. Treatment and homework formats.

A. Abbreviated Data Sheets for Session 5

Phase 1. Pretest. "Say words you can think of that have something to do specifically with the Renaissance" (5 minutes). Start time and end time were recorded, and words generated were listed and total reported to RR.

Phase 2. Demonstration. "This time I want you to write and then say words relating to the Renaissance" (5 minutes). Start time and end time were recorded, and words generated were listed and total reported to RR.

Phase 3. Practice. "Now we are going to practice writing and saying. We are going to use a new category. This time come up with words that relate to drama and dance. I will help you, but we will not go to a new word until you have said the one you have written" (25 minutes). Start time and end time were recorded, and words generated were listed and total reported to RR.

Phase 4. Posttest. "It's time to go back to Renaissance words. Remember your pen is now available. Use it if you need to. But we are trying to SAY these words" (5 minutes). Start time and end time were recorded, and words generated were listed and total reported to RR.

Phase 5. Conversation. "Let's talk about what you watched during this week's Olympics. Your pen is there to help you if you need it" (5 minutes). Start time and end time were recorded and words generated were listed and total reported to RR.

B. Homework (data from Week 10, Day 4)

Topic: Words that could be associated with WATER

Assignment: On each of 5 days this week, write 10 terms associated with the above topic. You can repeat words from the previous day if you wish. After you write each word, attempt to say it.* Evaluate your response as correct or incorrect. If you have not produced the word in 10 seconds, move on.

Term	Okay?	Term	Okay?
kayak	X	bikini	—
paddle	—	trunks	—
glacier	X	shower	X
iceberg	—	lather	X
hockey	—	bubble	—

---

*Originally, RR was asked to record the amount of time it took him to say each word. This proved too cumbersome for him, and he asked to be relieved of that responsibility.

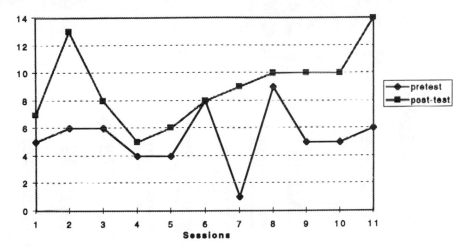

Figure 3–3. Phases 1 and 4 compared across sessions.

B. Pre- and Postcomparisons Across Sessions (Phase 1 versus Phase 4)

Figure 3–3 plots Phase 1 and 4 comparisons for each of the 11 sessions. Consistently higher performances were generated in Phase 4. RR produced approximately twice as many spoken words (spontaneously or assisted with writing) in the posttreatment phases. Pretreatment phases were variable, especially in the middle training sessions. The abnormally low performance in Session 7 pretest was probably because of RR's determination to name cleaning products (i.e., proper nouns), rather than to explore the larger corpus of instruments and generic words related to cleaning, which considerably limited the relevant semantic pool. He relaxed his self-imposed criterion in Phase 4 of this session. It should be noted that typically only about half of the words generated either in speaking or in writing in Phase 1 or Phase 2 showed up in posttesting, indicating that he was generating words from a larger semantic pool than he could come up with at any one time.

C. Within Treatment Performance

Figure 3–4 shows RR's word generation successes within each session. These data are relatively constant across sessions, with RR producing the largest number of words in the aberrant session 7. Largely, the data support the notion that all of the categories chosen for word generation presented similar ease (or difficulty) of access and once again support the notion of RR's largely intact access to his lexicon through writing.

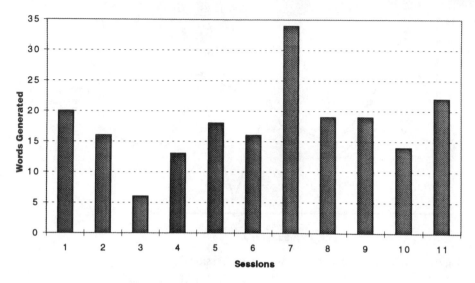

Figure 3–4. Performance during training phases for all sessions (Phase 3).

Because the categories selected for the naming activities covered a variety of more or less challenging topics and had the potential for evoking rare words and proper nouns, they had the potential for being more difficult than simply naming animals or words that begin with a designated alphabet letter. For example, here is a sampling of the variety of words RR generated during the treatment period. Each word was drawn from the stimulus category used on a different day. They are presented in order of sessions: "Buddha, Ukraine, Grand Canyon, spine, Isadora, hurricane, paprika, vacation, threatened, eyebrow."

An important change in RR's performance was that during these training sessions, RR increasingly made phonemic paraphasic errors, previously rare in both his discourse and clinical naming work. He recognized them as well, and largely was able to correct them. This suggests either that RR was permitting himself to make a few mistakes or that he was actually getting closer, somehow, to his phonological lexicon. In either case, as phonemic paraphasias provided more clues to listeners than did silence, they could be counted on to facilitate conversational interaction.

D. Conversation

Figure 3–5 depicts the number of substantive words that were spoken spontaneously or in conjunction with writing during the 5-minute conversation that ended each session. Data are presented for 9 of the 11

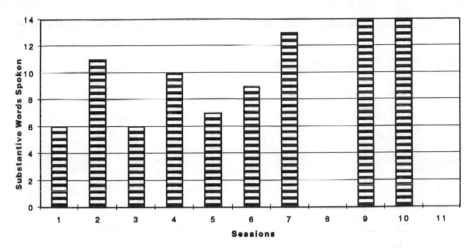

Figure 3–5. Number of substantive words spoken in each session's conversation (Phase 4).

sessions. This figure shows an increasing number of spoken words over the course of the sessions, suggesting that he was communicating more effectively in these timed conversations (possibly talking at a more normal rate or revising less frequently). A very interesting aspect of this increased efficiency is that, as these sessions went on, RR sometimes wrote only an initial letter, which facilitated his being able to say it. Occasionally, he simply reached forward with a pencil and in the process retrieved the word.

E. Homework

Figure 3–6 plots the mean number of homework words written and correctly said over 10 of the 11 weeks of this treatment, according to RR's own analysis of his successes and failures at word retrieval. Again, the data indicate a small, but growing effect. What is of interest here is that these mean data were accompanied by more consistent daily performance over the course of the treatment. That is, his variability was decreasing. It should again be noted that RR is his own worst critic in tasks such as these, in which he could choose to practice particularly pesky proper nouns and also exercise his tendency to judge anything but perfect production as "incorrect."

F. Other Measures

1. **Formal measure (WAB).** Near the end of this course of treatment, the WAB was readministered. At this last testing session, a WAB

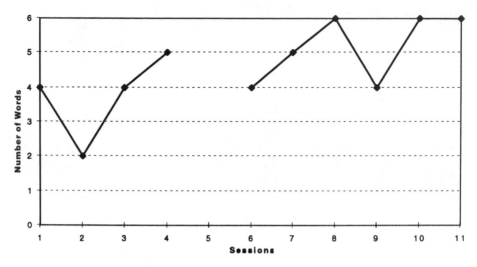

Figure 3–6. Mean number of words generated during homework sessions.

AQ of 71.8 (versus 62.8) was obtained. He continued to display conduction aphasia. This gain of 9 points exceeded the standard error of measurement (5 points) and is considered to be a significant improvement. It is noteworthy that RR's greatest gains were in naming (47 versus 73) and auditory comprehension (148 versus 179), respectively. It is of interest that his single word comprehension went from 47 of 60 to 55 of 60.

2. **Outcomes measure.** As suggested earlier, given his writing strategy RR's status as a functional communicator was never in question. Baseline assessments using measures such as Communicative Activities in Daily Living (CADL) and American Speech-Language-Hearing Association (ASHA)/Functional Assessment of Communicative Skills (FACS) for Adults would have produced performances that were near ceiling and largely useless for assessing the utility of this treatment. However, had this been earlier in the course of RR's recovery and had I been seeking third-party reimbursement, my report would have included something to the effect that: "In 11 sessions of therapy, RR has doubled his ability to say words independently using treatment activities that were generalizable to conversation, and therefore presumably to making his needs known and to providing information to others."

And in the face of his progress, I would seek, but would not be optimistic about receiving, reauthorization for further treatment.

All of the following observations of RR's change as a result of his treatment, however, suggest a positive functional outcome in his case.

a. Decreased use (but certainly not abandonment) of the notepads on which he wrote words that he could not say. RR reported that he was simply not having to resort to writing as frequently.

b. Decreased reliance on paper and pen as observed by two clinicians in RR's group therapy sessions. Three months following the conclusion of this brief treatment, RR used speech alone, with no supporting written substantive words, during a 20-minute conversation with two clinicians.

c. Self-reported increase in ability to communicate in Portuguese, with no deleterious effects on subsequent use of English.

d. Increasing appearance of target-related paraphasic errors in his speech.

This treatment was actually part of a research protocol and RR was not billed. However, it should be noted that had RR been billed at the ongoing rates of our clinic, the out-of-pocket cost would have been approximately $650.00.

VIII. DISCUSSION

A. General Comments

Despite all of the clinical interventions that RR has received to date, including the strategy described here, RR continues to struggle with his very unusual aphasic impairment. Nonetheless, there is little doubt that clinical intervention, coupled with his own intense motivation, interest, and self-discipline, contributed substantially to his improvement. What has not been addressed in this chapter is RR's unswerving belief that one of the most critical elements in his own survival as an aphasic person has been his contact with other aphasic persons through his involvement in aphasia groups. In a recently published popular article he completed with the help of his aphasia group and clinicians, he stated that he did not recover until he met other people who had aphasia. Certainly the large picture of recovery from aphasia and living as fully as one can despite its presence must take more than just one-on-one clinical intervention into account.

I am amazed by both RR's commitment and his progress. I continue to work with him, primarily because it is such a pleasure and a challenge to be a part of his world.

B. Alternatives

The autocue approach that was patterned on Nickels' work (1992) was highly relevant and largely effective as a first step. However, it failed to provide a mechanism for transfer to language use outside the clinic. To facilitate that transfer, there were few leads available in the literature, and I was not inventive enough to develop a less cumbersome and intellectually taxing approach than the one I described here. The literature does suggest that there might be ways to improve RR's written sentence production. Another patient's (AE's) treatment, as described by Mitchum et al. (1993) is certainly encouraging in that regard. RR and I have discussed the possibility of adapting their methods for our future work, and at some point, we will probably attempt it. But the major item on RR's agenda continues to be improving his speech production.

We are again doing some basic autocue work, now with vowels, coupled with a lot of rather old fashioned, but currently useful work of observing his speech sound making attempts in a mirror. (It is interesting that RR only recently has been able to make the connection between what he sees himself doing in a mirror and what he is apparently saying. I am not sure how to interpret this, but my best guess is that his phonological awareness simply continues to grow.) We know that the approach is successful for elicited word generation, but failed to generalize to more spontaneous word retrieval. Therefore, once a few more vowels are in place, we will attempt a version of the strategy reported here, but with emphasis on vowel-initial word retrieval.

C. Hindsight

In retrospect, would I do this form of treatment with RR again? The answer is yes—but elaborating it with the modifications I made during the course of the treatment from its outset. The approach did generalize to his daily use to some extent, and I have not yet found a suitable alternative approach to managing his phonological difficulties. Perhaps more to the point, would RR have been willing to do this form of treatment again? I have asked him, and his answer is yes.

IX. CONCLUSIONS

RR's problems are uncommon, but then to some extent every aphasic individual's problems are unique and govern clinical solutions. In RR's case, the decision making involved in RR's treatment from its inception also involved some general principles. The more important ones include:

- To the extent possible, involve the aphasic individual in choosing a course of action. In RR's case, we worked on the problem that bothered him the most. Additionally, the method we employed had no chance of success unless he understood it. Therefore, RR was constantly apprised of the rationale that underlay his particular treatment.

- Ensure that the aphasic individual takes as much responsibility for his or her own treatment as he or she can manage. For this reason, homework was an important component of the procedure used with RR.

- Attend to the aphasic individual's strengths and weaknesses and try to balance treatment between them. For RR, this meant focusing on deficit of impaired phonological access—but in a way that provided him with a strategy for manipulating it that was in keeping with his intellectual abilities and his motivation.

- Maintain flexibility. When clinical methods are unsuccessful, be prepared to change or modify them. In RR's treatment, the autocue approach provided a good beginning, but its failure to generalize motivated us to build upon it with the successful brief treatment that came next. I have also tried to indicate where changes were made on the basis of RR's response to the treatment.

X. ACKNOWLEDGMENTS

This work was supported in part by National Multipurpose Research and Training Center Grant DC-01409 from the National Institute on Deafness and Other Communicative Disorders. I thank Pelagie M. Beeson, Ph.D., for her help in conducting these therapy sessions, to Amy Ramage, M.S., and Shannon Bryant, M.S., for their previous work with RR, and Shannon Noga, our student clinician, for the last phase of this work. Most sincere gratitude goes to RR, for his dedication to this project, and for bettering the conditions of others with aphasia through his personal involvement in research and his development of aphasia groups.

XI. REFERENCES

Assal, G., Buttet, J., & Jolivet, R. (1981). Dissociations in aphasia: A case report. *Brain and Language, 13,* 223–240.

Berndt, R., Mitchum, D., Haendiges, A., & Sandson, J. (1997). Verb retrieval in aphasia, 1: Characterizing single word impairments. *Brain and Language, 56,* 68–106.

Bub, D., & Kertesz, A. (1982). Evidence of lexicographic processing in a patient with preserved written over oral single word naming. *Brain, 105,* 697–717.

Caramazza, A., Berndt, R., & Basili, A. (1983). The selective impairment phonological processing: A case study. *Brain and Language, 18,* 128–174.

Caramazza, A., & Hillis, A. (1991). Lexical organization of nouns and verbs in the brain. *Nature, 349,* 788–790.

Ellis, A., Miller, D., & Sin, G. (1983). Wernicke's aphasia and normal language processing: A case study in cognitive neuropsychology. *Cognition, 15,* 111–144.

Farah, M. J., & Wallace, M. A. (1992). Semantically bounded anomia: Implications for neural implementation of naming. *Neuropsychologia, 30*(7), 692–621.

Helm-Estabrooks, N. (1992). *Aphasia diagnostic profiles.* Chicago, IL: Riverside Publishing Co.

Hier, D., & Mohr, J. (1977). Incongruous oral and written naming: Evidence for a subdivision of the syndrome Wernicke's aphasia. *Brain and Language, 4,* 115–126.

Kay, J., Lesser, L., & Coltheart, M. (1992). *PALPA: Psycholinguistic Assessments of Language Processing in Aphasia.* East Sussex, UK: Lawrence Erlbaum.

Kertesz, I. (1992). *Western Aphasia Battery.* New York: Grune and Stratton.

Kremin, H. (1987). Is there more than ah-oh-oh? Alternative strategies for writing and repeating lexically. In M. Coltheart, G. G. Satori, & R. Job (Eds.), *The cognitive neuropsychology of language.* London: LEA, Ltd.

Levine, D., Calvanio, R., & Popovics, X. (1982). Language in the absence of inner speech. *Neuropsychologia, 20,* 391–409.

Lesser, R. (1989). Some issues in the neuropsychological rehabilitation of anomia. In X. Seron & G. Deloche (Eds.), *Cognitive approaches to neuropsychological rehabilitation.* Hillsdale, NJ: Lawrence Erlbaum.

Lowell, S., Beeson, P., & Holland, A. (1995). The efficacy of a semantic cueing procedure on naming performance of adults with aphasia. Clinical Aphasiology Proceedings. *American Journal of Speech-Language Pathology, 4,* 109–114.

Mitchum, C., Berndt, R., & Haendiges, S. (1993). Model-guided treatment to improve written sentence production: A case study. *Aphasiology, 7*(1),71–109.

Nickels, L. (1992). The autocue? Self-generated phonemic cues in the treatment of a disorder of reading and naming. *Cognitive Neuropsychology, 9,* 155–182.

Patterson, K., & Shewell, C. (1987). Speak and spell: Dissociations and word class effects. In M. Coltheart, G. G. Satori, & R. Job (Eds.), *The cognitive neuropsychology of language.* London: LEA, Ltd.

Raymer, A., & Berndt, R. (1996). Reading lexically without semantics: Evidence from patients with probable Alzheimer's disease. *Journal of the International Neuropsychological Society, 2,* 340–349.

Ross, R. (1995). Aphasia groups: A view from the inside. *Advance Magazine.*

Shelton, J., & Weinrich, M. (in press). Further evidence of a dissociation between output phonological and orthographic lexicons: A case study. *Cognitive Neuropsychology.*

Warrington, E. K., & Shallice, T. (1984). Category specific semantic impairments. *Brain, 101,* 829–854.

Weinrich, M., Shelton, J., & McCall, D. (1997a). Remediating production of tense morphology improved verb production in chronic aphasia. *Brain and Language, 58*(1), 23.

Weinrich, M., Shelton, J. R., & Cox, D. (1997b). Generalization from single sentence to multi-sentence production in severely aphasic patients. *Brain and Language, 58*(2), 327.

Zingeser, L., & Berndt, R. (1988). Grammatical class and context effects in a case of pure anomia: Implications for a model of language processing. *Cognitive Neuropsychology, 5,* 473–516

CHAPTER

4

A "Cognitive" Approach to Treatment of an Aphasic Patient

NANCY HELM-ESTABROOKS, Sc.D.

I. BACKGROUND

A. The Issue of Cognition and Aphasia

Cognition and language are not separate entities. Instead, language is one aspect of cognition, along with attention and concentration, learning and memory, visuospatial abilities, and executive functions. The extent to which aspects of cognition, other than language, may be impaired in aphasic patients is unresolved and continues to be an issue for continuing research (Hamsher, 1991). The study of cognition in aphasia is difficult because most tests of intelligence are language-based, making them invalid for use with aphasic patients. Studies using "nonverbal" tests of various cognitive abilities have produced mixed evidence of a functional relationship between aphasia and nonverbal intelligence. A 1995 study (Helm-Estabrooks, Bayles, Ramage, & Bryant) of "nonverbal" cognitive performance and aphasia severity in 32 nonglobal aphasic patients found no significant relationship between the two. Some severely aphasic patients performed quite well on tests of attention, visuoperception/construction, memory, and executive functions and some patients with relatively milder aphasia performed poorly.

The issue of the relationship between cognition and aphasia is not inconsequential. The extent to which cognitive skills may be spared or impaired in aphasic patients is pivotal to treatment of their aphasia. At its most basic level, therapy requires the ability to attend and concentrate and memory is critical to all learning. Integrity of visuoperceptual skills is needed for processing many treatment materials, and, finally, executive skills are required if a patient is to develop and implement ways to communicate in unique situations despite aphasia. Ultimately, patients with aphasia must compensate for their language problems through a dynamic process of problem solving that requires them to assess communicative situations, generate plans for conveying target messages and then put these plans into effect. Determining levels of competence in all areas of cognition appears to be fundamental to aphasia treatment.

B. Cognitive Versus Linguistic Approaches to Aphasia Treatment

Linguistic approaches to treatment of aphasia assume that a patient's problems lie exclusively in the domain of language, but some aphasiologists (e.g., Goldstein, 1948; Martin, 1981; Wepman, 1972) have argued that language cannot be isolated from other aspects of cognition. In fact, Martin defines aphasia as "the reduction, because of brain damage, of the efficiency of action and interaction of the cognitive processes which support language behavior" (p. 148). It would appear from our 1995 study, however, that some aphasic patients demonstrate relative sparing of other aspects of cognition and that therapy can be focused directly on language. For those in whom other areas of cognition are impaired, treatment of the communication disorder may, necessarily, involve treatment of skills within those cognitive domains. In fact, Van Mourik, Vershaeve, Boon, and Harskamp (1992) stated that "patients with impairment of basic cognitive skills should be treated non-verbally to create a sufficient basis for language-oriented treatment and communication strategies" (p. 497). Little attention has been given to developing and testing such therapies.

In this chapter, I describe an aphasic stroke patient with problems in several cognitive domains that were addressed during a short course (10, 1-hour sessions in 10 weeks) of therapy.

II. THE PATIENT

A. Biography

Mr. B was a 57-year-old, right-handed man with a Bachelor of Science in engineering and a Master's degree in business administration who had been an executive with a large manufacturing company at the time of his stroke. He was married, had two grown children of his own and one stepdaughter. Before his stroke, he had played golf and traveled extensively. At the time of this treatment he enjoyed photography, movies, card playing, listening to music, and dining out.

B. Medical History

Mr. B had a history of bleeding peptic ulcers and hypertension, and in July 1992 suffered a left intracerebral hemorrhage. He was unresponsive for several weeks and then required a craniotomy for the bleeding. About two weeks later, he awoke with dysphagia, global aphasia, right hemiparesis, and loss of right peripheral vision. Around this time he developed a seizure disorder. Over the next 2 years, he regained some language skills, and was no longer globally aphasic although he remained densely hemiplegic. During an automobile trip in December 1994, he had sudden onset of worsening aphasia. He was admitted to a hospital, but reports there failed to document the basis for the event. In May 1995, Mr. B broke his pelvis when he fell during a seizure. In September 1995, he again fell during a seizure and broke his hip. An unenhanced CT scan performed in May 1996 showed a large area of encephalomalacia in the left basal ganglia and frontal lobe along with an old right occipital lobe infarct and a lacune in the right corona radiata. His drug regimen in 1996 included two anticonvulsants (Neurontin and Lamictal) and two antihypertensive medications (Triamterene and Normodyne).

C. Previous Management

In the 9 months following his 1992 stroke, Mr. B received speech/language therapy at a facility in his home city. Reports as to the nature and intensity of this therapy were not available but, initially, he was described as having "severely impaired communication skills, unawareness of overlearned environmental sounds, marked deficits in visual perception and integration, and a high level of frustration." On discharge, he was said to have made "tremendous progress in all areas" but no test data were provided to document these improvements. In December 1994, he and his wife moved to Tucson, AZ.

In January 1995 he was tested at the Aphasia Clinic at the University of Arizona with the *Aphasia Diagnostic Profiles* (ADP, Helm-Estabrooks, 1992). His aphasia severity standard score was 99 (47th percentile). Auditory comprehension (ss = 12; 75th percentile) was significantly better than lexical retrieval (ss = 7; 16th percentile) and repetition (ss = 8; 25th percentile). His aphasia profile classified him as borderline fluent aphasia. His best average phrase length was longer than that of typical of nonfluent syndromes such as Broca's aphasia and shorter than that seen in fluent syndromes such as Wernicke's aphasia. His course of therapy included 23 weekly sessions of individual and group therapy, between February and April, 1995. Individual therapy involved various cuing techniques to elicit key words and phrases. Homework consisted of questions such as "What is your favorite color?" that he was supposed to answer by typing responses on his computer. Response to these approaches appears to have been poor and he was said to be "slow to complete his homework." Group therapy encouraged a total communication approach of using words, gestures, and drawing to convey messages. No posttesting was performed at semester's end. In the fall of 1995 Mr. B attended two group sessions before entering the hospital for a hip repair. Not surprisingly, he was described in his clinic record as being somewhat depressed. He re-entered the University of Arizona Aphasia Center program in January 1996.

III. APPRAISAL

A. Rationale

For several reasons, I suspected that Mr. B might have other notable cognitive deficits in addition to his aphasia: (1) his medical history of cerebral hemorrhage, coma, and craniotomy; (2) early reports that he had attention and visual perceptual problems; (3) his bilateral lesions; (4) his poor response at our clinic to more traditional "linguistic" therapy approaches; and (5) his recent exposure to general anesthesia for hip surgeries. To determine the presence and extent of other deficits, I administered a "nonverbal" cognitive test battery of tests/tasks selected to tap a variety of cognitive skills (see following descriptions). To determine the current status of his aphasia, I readministered the Aphasia Diagnostic Profiles.

B. Assessment Methods

1. **Nonverbal Cognitive Test Battery.** The cognitive battery consisted of five "nonverbal" tasks and tests used in our 1995 study (Helm-Estabrooks, et al., 1995) as measures of attention and concentration, memory, visuoperception and construction, and executive functions. These tasks were as follows:

   a. **Clock drawing/setting to command.** According to Freedman et al. (1994), the ability to draw a clock and set the hands at "10 after 11" requires several cognitive functions including: (1) ability to internally represent the visuospatial features of a clock; (2) visuoperceptual and visuomotor processes for translating the mental representation into a motor program for drawing and for guiding the spatial layout of component features; (3) right and left hemiattention to assure that clock features are represented accurately in both sides of space; working memory to temporarily hold and process the information; and (5) executive functions for planning, organization, and making corrections. A specially devised scoring system for this task yields a total high score of 37.

   b. **A modified version of the *Wisconsin Card Sort Test* (WCST) (Nelson, 1976).** This test assesses ability to establish and shift conceptual sets. The subject must match a series of cards to four target cards displaying stimuli that vary in color, shape, and number. The sorting principles are never stated explicitly but must be deduced from the examiner's feedback as to whether the sorting response was right or wrong. For example, the first sort should be according to color. If a patient sorts first by number or shape, he or she is told "no" until the switch is made to color which is reinforced with "yes." After the subject has produced six consecutive correct responses, the sorting principle is changed abruptly ("no") and the subject must discover the new principle. Highest possible score = 6 sets.

   c. *Wechsler Memory Scale—Revised* (WMS-R) (Wechsler, 1987) **Visual paired associates subtests.** In this test, six colors are paired with six abstract designs. The object of the test is for the subject to learn and subsequently recall the associations. First, each design is presented with its associated color. Then, each design is presented without its matching color. The examinee must indicate by pointing to the associated color depicted on a card displaying all six colors. Subjects are given up to three learning trials to master the pairings. Highest score = 18.

d. **WMS-R Figural memory subtest.** This is a multiple-choice test of visuoperception and visual memory for abstract designs. The first item requires the subject to study a design and then identify it from a field of three. In subsequent items the subject must identify three remembered items from fields of nine. Highest score = 10.

e. **WMS-R Visual memory span subtest.** In this test of immediate memory, the subject is presented with a card displaying a random array of green squares. The examiner begins by touching two squares. The subject watches and then repeats this pattern. Another pattern of two then is presented and if the subject successfully imitates at least one of the two presentations, the pointing span is increased to three and so on up to seven consecutive squares. Highest score = 14.

2. **Cognitive Scoring.** *The highest overall score for the cognitive battery is 85.* In the study by Helm-Estabrooks et al. (1995), a group of 31 normal elders earned a mean score of 69 (s.d. = 13.2) and a group of 32 aphasic (nonglobal) stroke patients with unilateral left hemisphere lesions earned a mean score of 53.63 (SD = 8.6; range = 31–69).

3. **Language Exam**

a. **Aphasia Diagnostic Profiles (Helm-Estabrooks, 1992).** This test was standardized on more than 300 individuals drawn from 42 centers across the United States and Canada. The average administration time is 45 minutes and the test yields profiles of aphasia severity, aphasia classification, alternative communication abilities, error types and behavior. ADP aphasia severity is based on standard scores earned on lexical retrieval (personal information, information units given in describing a pictured scene, and confrontation naming), auditory comprehension, and repetition. Lexical retrieval and auditory comprehension are given double weight in determining aphasia severity, which can be expressed as a percentile rank.

4. **Determination of Functional Needs.** To identify some of Mr. B's "functional" problems, his wife was given an informal questionnaire and asked to make a list of her husband's most pressing difficulties and needs of everyday living.

C. Assessment Results

1. **Cognitive Battery.** On the nonlinguistic cognitive battery, Mr B earned an overall score of 22/85. This score is more than three standard deviations below the mean for (nonglobal) aphasic patients and therefore represents significant cognitive deficits. Individual test scores recorded in January 1996 are shown below.

Cognitive Battery Scores Earned on 1/96	
Clock drawing/setting	= 12/37
WCST (shortened version)	= 5/6
WMS-R Figural memory	= 2/10
WMS-R Visual paired associates	= 0/18
WMS-R Visual memory span	= 3/14
Total Score	= 22/85
Mean for nonglobal aphasic patients	= 54/85 (s.d. = 8.6)
Mean for normal elders	= 66/85 (s.d. = 13.2)

2. **Aphasia Test.** Readministration of the ADP on 1/26/96 showed a significant worsening of Mr. B's aphasia severity (AS) since 1/17/95. Significant changes in ADP performance are determined according to standard scores with nonoverlapping confidence intervals based on standard errors of measurement (SEM). (The SEM is simply the number of points that, when added to and subtracted from the obtained score, provides the upper and lower limits of the confidence range within a certain probability (ADP Manual, Helm-Estabrooks, 1992). Mr. B's AS standard score had dropped from 99 (47th percentile) to 92 (30th percentile). Examination of modality-specific scores showed that auditory comprehension was responsible for AS score decline, with a dip from a standard score of 12 (75th percentile) in 1/95 to 9 (37th percentile) in 1/96. Lexical retrieval was unchanged from 1/95 to 1/96, with an earned standard

score of 7 (16th percentile) on both occasions. His repetition standard score of 8 (25th percentile) also was unchanged from 1/95 to 1/96. Another measure of performance on the ADP is alternative communication, which is a composite of scores on subtests of reading, writing, elicited gestures, and singing. On 1/96 Mr. B's alternative communication standard score of 98 (45th percentile) was significantly better than his 1/95 score of 92 (30th percentile). Singing was the modality that had improved, by three standard scores (34 percentile points). His ability to read, write, and gesture had not changed significantly. His 1/96 behavioral profile ratings earned him a standard score of 90 (25th percentile), which was not significantly worse than his 1/95 score of 93 (32nd percentile). The ADP scores from these two testing dates follow:

Mr. B's Aphasia Diagnostic Profiles		
ADP Scores	**1/17/95**	**1/26/96**
Overall Aphasia Severity	**47th %ile (ss= 99)**	**30th %ile (ss= 92)***
Auditory comprehension	75th %ile (ss=12)	37th %ile (ss=9)*
Lexical retrieval	16th %ile (ss=7)	16th %ile (ss=7)
Repetition	25th %ile (ss=8)	25th %ile (ss=8)
Alternative communication	30th %ile (ss=92)	45th %ile (ss=98)**
Behavior	32nd %ile (ss=93)	25th %ile (ss=90)

*Significant decline
**Significant improvement

3. **Functional Questionnaire.** The functional problems listed by Mrs. B. included:

   a. Coming up with the right words when he wants.

   b. Frustration when he can not make himself understood.

   c. Wanting to read and write.

   d. Bumping into things on the right side around the house and in the neighborhood.

   e. Not seeing food that is on the right side of his plate.

   f. Not driving the golf cart because he is not seeing everything.

IV. DIAGNOSIS

A. The Disorders

1. **Nonlinguistic Cognitive Deficits.** The results of the nonverbal cognitive testing indicated that Mr. B had notable problems in visuoperception and construction, and working memory and learning as indicated by his poor scores on clock drawing/setting, figural memory, visual memory span, and visual paired associates. In contrast, his WCST performance suggested relative preservation of the ability to establish and shift mental sets, a skill thought to be an important aspect of executive functions.

2. **Language Deficits.** Mr. B's ADP aphasia severity standard score of 92 (30th percentile) indicated that he had relatively severe aphasia. Auditory comprehension was significantly better than lexical retrieval. Repetition ability was not significantly worse than auditory comprehension nor significantly better than lexical retrieval. His standard scores for confrontation naming, average best phrase length, auditory comprehension, and repetition were in keeping with a classification of borderline fluent aphasia associated with relatively poor auditory comprehension and repetition. His alternative communication scores indicated that reading, writing, gesturing, and singing, although quite impaired, were significantly better than the skills that relied more heavily on verbal encoding and decoding.

3. **Functional Problems.** Mr. B's everyday problems, as reported by his wife, were in keeping with his formal test performance. His difficulty in "coming up with the right words when he wants" was reflected in his poor performance (16th percentile) on ADP tests of lexical retrieval. Mr. B also had indicated that he wanted to improve his reading and writing. On the ADP, reading and writing are briefly assessed with a questionnaire that requires the patient to write personal information such as name and address and circle correct answers from multiple choice questions about such matters as employment status. Compared with some other standardized aphasia tests, the ADP examines reading and writing in a practical, but perfunctory, fashion. Even so, Mr. B. scored only at the 37th percentile on writing and the 63rd percentile on reading, clearly indicative of marked deficits for a former executive with a graduate degree. His frustration as reported by his wife was noted also during testing. Other behaviors shown in the test situation included some impulsivity, emotional lability, self-deprecation, discouragement,

and anxiety. All of these were reflected in his ADP behavioral profile score, which was at the 25th percentile. In addition, cognitive testing picked up the everyday visual perceptual problems Mr. B displayed as he attempted to carry out certain daily activities and negotiate within his environment. His clock drawing was poor (12/37), as was his performance on tests with visual perception and memory demands (figural memory = 2/10, visual memory span = 3/14, and visual paired associates = 0/18).

B. Other Considerations

Mr. B's performance on language and nonlinguistic cognitive tests was in keeping with his problems with everyday functional activities. But, it is important to consider the impact of his medications and ongoing medical problems (including seizures and surgery) on his test performance, mood, and previous response to therapy. Neurontin, Lamictal, Triameterene, and Normodyne are powerful drugs that, together, affect virtually every body system and metabolic pathway. In addition, on May 14, 1995 and again in September of that year, Mr. B underwent surgery with general anesthesia for a broken pelvis and then a hip. The effects of general anaesthesia on the mental processes of persons with compromised brain tissue should always be of concern, although his wife did not report a change in his language skills and mentation subsequent to surgery. But, from her description and that of others, it is clear that he was psychologically depressed and discouraged by his medical problems. Finally, in thinking about factors that may have negatively affected his performance, we must consider the recurrence of seizures despite anticonvulsant medications.

V. PROGNOSIS

A. Prognostic Indicators

1. **Positive Prognostic Indicators.** Mr. B's indicators for treatment response included the following:

   a. He was a relatively young age (57 years).

   b. He probably had high premorbid intelligence, having earned an advanced college degree.

   c. He apparently had the interpersonal skills necessary for functioning as a company executive.

   d. He had a lifelong interest in new learning and adventures.

e. He had a supportive spouse and family.

f. He had no financial worries.

g. He lived in a climate that allowed him to be out and about throughout the year.

h. He expressed a desire to improve his communication skills.

2. **Negative Prognostic Indicators.** Mr. B's negative indicators for treatment response included the following:

   a. He was 3½ years postonset of an intracerebral hemorrhage.

   b. He had extensive brain damage that included a large left cerebral lesion with both cortical and basal ganglia involvement as well as a right occipital lesion and a right corona radiata lacune.

   c. His hemorrhage resulted in 2 weeks of "coma" before a craniotomy was performed.

   d. His auditory comprehension had declined significantly between 1/95 and 1/96.

   e. He had shown little improvement in verbal skills and remained significantly aphasic despite a course of linguistically oriented treatment.

   f. His performance on nonlinguistic cognitive tests indicated notable visual perceptual, learning, memory, and planning problems.

   g. He had felt discouraged and depressed for about 5 months before beginning this new phase of treatment.

B. Expected Outcomes

At 3½ years postonset, Mr. B was well beyond the period during which we might expect significant spontaneous recovery from his aphasia. Furthermore, his response to linguistic treatment at 2½ years postonset was poor; he remained very restricted in his ability to produce propositional speech and his auditory comprehension declined significantly between 1995 and 1996. It appeared that continued efforts to improve language in a "head-on" manner would not be effective. If Van Mourik and colleagues (1992) are correct in advising that nonlinguistic cognitive problems should be addressed before linguistic-oriented treatments are initiated, then we would expect a more "cognitive" approach to treatment to produce better results than previous language therapy attempts. This nontraditional approach, also, would be in keeping with Martin's (1981) belief that language behavior is supported by the action and interaction of other cognitive processes.

VI. FOCUSING THE TREATMENT

A. Rationale

The rationale for addressing Mr. B's cognitive deficits in therapy is that his score of 22/85 on the cognitive battery indicated severe problems in some nonlinguistic cognitive domains. Furthermore, he had not responded to linguistic approaches to aphasia rehabilitation. It seemed that a program directed at improving his cognitive problems might yield better results or at least prepare the ground for future attempts to improve his propositional speech.

B. Methods

Mr. B was treated for 10, 1-hour sessions of cognitive therapy approximately weekly between February and April 1996. He was always given home assignments, requiring 1–2 hours of work, and he always completed these assignments although not without errors. All homework was reviewed with Mr. B and he was helped with error correction before new tasks were introduced. In addition to this individualized treatment, he attended 12 group therapy sessions with three other men and a clinician. The foci of these sessions were current events, places of interest, personally relevant issues, and hypothetical situations.

Individual sessions of cognitive therapy targeted the domains and tasks in the order of the following list.

1. Attention and Concentration Tasks:

a. Cancellation of target lines, numbers, letters, and symbols.

b. Repeated and alternating graphomotor patterns.

c. Trail making with numbers, letters, and numbers and letters.

2. Visual Memory Tasks:

a. Memory for abstract designs.

b. Memory for pictured objects.

3. Counting, Number Fact, Judgment, and Estimation Tasks:

   a. Counting using dots.

   b. Explicit number facts with visual cues and multiple choices, such as, "How many minutes in an hour?"

   c. Rank ordering same-size pictures of items according to real object size and weight.

   d. Rank ordering items according to estimated cost.

   e. Estimating the cost of items.

4. Visuoperception and Construction Tasks:

   a. Visual matching of abstract designs.

   b. Visual judgments of "odd-man-out" using abstract designs.

   c. Completion of incomplete pictures.

   d. Clock drawing and setting.

   e. Identifying geographic locations (e.g., cities, rivers, countries) on maps.

5. Semantic Knowledge Tasks:

   a. Linking pictured objects according to functional relationships, such as camera and film.

   b. Identification of items according to function, properties, color, and sounds.

   c. Sorting pictured items according to semantic categories, such as fruits, motorized vehicles. First, the sorting principles were given to him; later, he had to identify the sorting principles.

   d. Semantic "odd-man-out," such as pelican, bat, cardinal, duck.

Many of these tasks were taken from the *Cognitive Linguistic Task Book* (Helm-Estabrooks, 1995). When Mr. B experienced difficulty with any task, it was simplified and then gradually made more complex until he could complete the original task. For example, symbol cancellation was carried out by asking Mr. B to cross out 29 target abstract symbols on a page displaying a random distribution of 112 occurrences of different abstract symbols. Mr. B was unable to do this task because he was "pulled" to tracing both target and nontarget symbols and showed neglect of the right side of the page. Using a Xerox machine, I enlarged the original page so that fewer, more widely spaced symbols were displayed. I then had him scan the symbols through a "window" cut in an index card, so that he could consider each separately. Using this approach, he was successful in "canceling" only the target symbols. I then slowly increased the field of targets and foils and faded the use of the "window" card until he could complete the original task.

VII. RESULTS

The within-treatment outcome measures were his ability to eventually complete each task in its unmodified form correctly and without assistance.

Improvement in Mr. B's cognitive-linguistic skills was measured through readministration of the cognitive battery, the ADP, and the functional questionnaire.

A. Cognitive Battery

On 5/12/96 Mr. B earned an overall score of 44/85 (approximately 1 standard deviation below the mean for aphasic patients). Individual test scores are contrasted with pretreatment scores below:

Mr. B's Cognitive Battery Scores		
	1/26/96 *Pretreatment*	*5/26/96* *Posttreatment*
Clock drawing/setting	= 12/37	28/37
WCST (shortened version)	= 5/6	1/6
WMS-R figural memory	= 2/10	5/10
WMS-R visual paired associates	= 0/18	4/18
WMS-R visual memory span	= 3/14	6/14
Total Score	**= 22/85**	**44/85**
Mean for nonglobal aphasia	= 54/85	
Mean for normal elders	= 66/85	

The astute reader will notice that, although Mr. B's overall score on the cognitive battery of 5/26/96 was 22 points higher than that of 1/26/96, his score declined on the WCST. This occurred because he attempted to outsmart the tester. After he had sorted the first category (color) correctly, receiving 6 successive "yes" reinforcements in a row, he was told "no" to indicate that he should try a different sorting strategy. He did switch, but after that, he anticipated the change after 5 correct sorts. Thus, he never again performed the 6 correct sorts necessary for him to earn additional credit.

B. Aphasia Diagnostic Profiles

The ADP was readministered on 5/26/96. The scores earned on this date are compared with those earned on 1/26/96 below.

Mr. B's Aphasia Diagnostic Profiles		
ADP Scores	*1/26/96*	*5/26/96*
Overall aphasia severity	*30th %ile*	*61st %ile*
	(ss=92)	*(ss=104)***
Auditory comprehension	37th %ile (ss=9)	95th %ile (ss=15)**
Lexical retrieval	16th %ile (ss=7)	16th %ile (ss=7)
Repetition	25th %ile (ss=8)	37th %ile (ss=9)
Alternative communication	45th %ile (ss=98)	37th %ile (ss=95)*
Behavior	25th %ile (ss=90)	42nd %ile (ss=97)

*Significant decline
**Significant improvement

As can be seen by examining these scores, Mr. B's overall aphasia severity improved a significant 31 percentile points. The modality most responsible for this change was auditory comprehension, which improved by 58 percentile points, although no specific treatment was given for auditory comprehension. Improvement in this area occurred secondary to work within other cognitive domains such as attention and concentration, memory, and semantic knowledge. This finding underscores the complexity of the language system and suggests that our treatments might well be directed at processes underlying comprehension of speech. His behavioral profile score also improved significantly. Finally, the significant decline in alternative communication scores was secondary to a drop in his reading performance as tested by circling answers on a questionnaire.

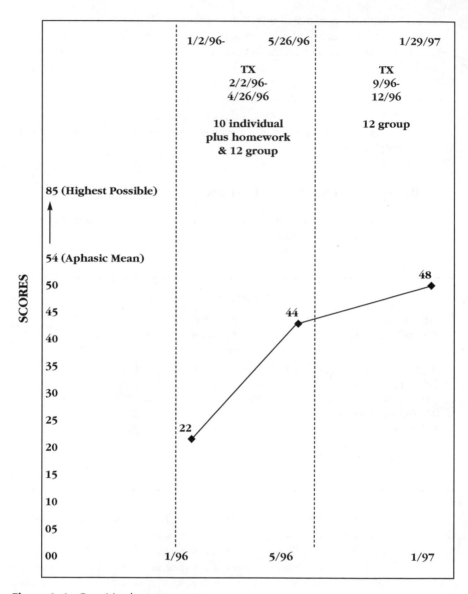

Figure 4–1. Cognitive battery scores

C. Functional Questionnaire

In the last weeks of therapy, Mrs. B was asked to note changes in her husband's everyday behavior. Here are the changes she listed.

- Saying "good night" instead of "bye."

- He's using more phrases and natural groups of words rather than one word; e.g., he said about his homework "I read it slowly and accurately."

- He drove the golf cart for the first time and did well.

- He cut up some vegetables and folded some laundry for the first time.

- He went bowling with us and kept score.

- He put his left sock on by himself for the first time.

The improvements seen in Mr. B's functional activities were not entirely those expected to result from aphasia therapy. Although changes were noted in his everyday communication, more changes occurred in other endeavors, particularly those that depended on his visuospatial and perceptual skills. These daily activities are more typically the concern of occupational therapy, which Mr. B. was no longer receiving. Certainly his reacquired ability to participate to some extent in family sports and to help with household chores had a positive effect on the overall quality of his (and his wife's) life.

VIII. FINAL RETESTING

Retesting was conducted 8 months after this course of treatment was completed. Mr. B had no treatment during the intervening summer months, but attended 12, 1-hour group sessions during the fall semester. On 1/29/97, Mr. B's overall score on the battery of cognitive tests was 48/85 (an increase of 4 points since 5/26/96). His ADP aphasia severity score was at the 63rd percentile (an insignificant gain of 2 percentile points), with auditory comprehension remaining at the 95th percentile. In Figures 4–1 and 4–2 the improvements made by Mr. B on cognitive and aphasia testing with 10 weekly sessions of cognitive-linguistic treatment are graphically depicted. These figures also illustrate the maintenance of gains over a subsequent 8 month period during which he only attended aphasia group sessions.

IX. DISCUSSION

A. Rationale

Although Jackson (1878) was the first to speak of an intellectual defect in association with aphasia in the English literature, Vignolo (1989)

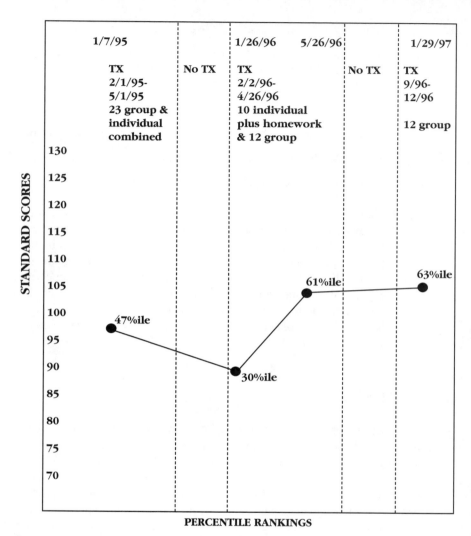

Figure 4–2. Aphasia diagnostic profile standard scores for aphasia severity.

pointed out that Paul Broca was the first to mention this association. Our research (Helm-Estabrooks et al., 1995) indicates that performance on an aphasia test is not significantly correlated with performance on non-verbal tests of cognitive functions, that is, knowing a person's aphasia test score will not predict how well they will perform on nonverbal cognitive tasks. Some severely aphasic patients perform quite well on them, with some more mildly aphasic patients performing poorly. For patients with nonverbal cognitive deficits as well as aphasia, clinical researchers such as Van Mourik et al. (1992) believe that treatment of these cognitive deficits must precede attempts to directly treat the communication problem. I concur. It is known that certain cognitive skills provide the underpinnings for language acquisition. These same skills may be necessary for successful rehabilitation of language following acquired aphasia. Certainly, functions such as attention and concentration, learning, and memory are basic to treatment response. And, ultimately, aphasic patients must have good problem-solving skills/ executive functions (planning, initiating and carrying out goal-directed activities) to make the best of their residual language skills.

The case presented here, Mr. B, had moderate aphasia and notable nonverbal cognitive deficits. He had not responded to an earlier course of direct language treatment. For that reason, I chose to spend the 10 hourly treatment sessions concentrating on nonverbal aspects of cognition. I supplemented these sessions with homework assignments, which he always carried out. His response to this treatment approach was good. He demonstrated significant changes in nonverbal cognitive and aphasia test performance (especially auditory comprehension) and in the functional skills reported by his wife. Further, these gains were maintained over the next 8 months. Since treating Mr. B, I have been able to obtain similar results with two other cognitively compromised aphasic patients who were past the period of greatest spontaneous recovery (5 months and 11 months). As with Mr. B, both individuals were premorbidly bright and in their 50s and, also like him, one had bilateral lesions. Both had responded poorly to linguistic treatment before I treated them with 7 sessions of therapy with homework. These cases support the opinion of Van Mourik et al. (1992) that in aphasia rehabilitation impairment of basic cognitive skills should be addressed before language treatments are undertaken.

B. Alternatives

The patient described in this chapter was not only aphasic, he displayed nonverbal cognitive problems. As stated earlier, cognition has at least five primary domains (attention/concentration, learning/memory, visuoperception/construction, language, and executive functions). In designing a treatment program to target these areas, I developed certain tasks. It is important to note, however, that successful completion of most clinical activities requires the use of several cognitive functions. Consider, for example, cancellation tasks such as crossing out target symbols from a randomly presented array. These tasks often are given to assess or improve concentration and attention. At the same time, however, they require visuoperceptual skills for discriminating the stimuli, working memory for remembering the aim of the task and the target stimulus, and motor skills for making crosses. Furthermore, use of spoken and written instructions engages the patient's language skills, although the clinician may be able to gesturally demonstrate the intent of the exercise. But, although most tasks tap multiple domains, some tasks predominately require one particular skill. For example, the ability to group stimuli according to some classifying principle, such as citrus fruits, relies heavily on semantic knowledge. In treating Mr. B, I targeted certain cognitive domains and worked with him on exercises that seemed to be heavily weighed towards those skills. Certainly, many other exercises or tasks might have done the same job. Compared with his poor response to linguistic-oriented therapy, his response to a short course of "cognitive" therapy was so good that I would have continued on that track, expanding the type and difficulty of tasks as he progressed.

C. Hindsight

If I could work with Mr. B again, I would obtain better pre- and post-therapy measures of his functional status, which are considered to be critical indicators of the effectiveness of therapy. Furthermore, given his reported history of "depression," I would administer a psychosocial scale that might provide insight into his moods, outlook, frustration levels, and so on before, during, and after treatment. (See Lyon in this text for such scales.) And, because aphasia and its concomitant problems are family problems, I would administer a psychosocial scale to his wife as well and, depending on the result, possibly recommend family counseling.

Certainly one uncontrolled variable in this case is that, during the time that I treated him, he also received group therapy. We have good evidence that group therapy alone did not enhance his test performance, but he probably should receive a course of cognitive therapy alone to test its independent effectiveness. The two other previously mentioned patients that I treated with a similar program received only individual cognitive treatment and responded comparably. This variable should be controlled for in future cases.

X. ACKNOWLEDGMENTS

The author wishes to thank Margaret Forbes, University of Pittsburgh, for her careful editing of this chapter. Dr. Helm-Estabrooks' work was supported by the National Institute for Deafness and Communication Disorders Grant

#DC01409 to the National Center for Neurogenic Communication Disorders at the University of Arizona.

XI. REFERENCES

Freedman, M., Leach, L., Kaplan, E., Winocur, G., Shulman, K., & Delis, D. (1994). *Clock drawing: A neuropsychological analysis.* New York: Oxford University Press.

Goldstein, K. (1948). *Language and language disturbances.* New York: Grune and Stratton.

Hamsher, K. (1991). Intelligence and aphasia. In M. T. Sarno (Ed.), *Acquired aphasia.* (pp. 339–372). New York: Academic Press.

Helm-Estabrooks, N. (1992). *Aphasia diagnostic profiles.* Chicago: Applied Symbolix.

Helm-Estabrooks, N. (1995). *Cognitive linguistic task book.* Sandwich, MA: Cape Cod Institute for Communication Disorders–Publishing Division.

Helm-Estabrooks, N., Bayles, K., Ramage, A., & Bryant, S. (1995). The relationship between cognitive performance and aphasia severity, age, and education: Females versus males. *Brain and Language, 51*(1)139–141.

Jackson, H. (1878). On affections of speech from disease of the brain. *Brain, 1,* 304–330

Martin, A. D. (1981). An examination of Wepman's thought centered therapy. In R. Chapey (Ed.), *Language intervention strategies in adult aphasia* (pp. 141–154). Baltimore: Williams and Wilkins.

Nelson, H. E. (1976). A modified card sorting test sensitive to frontal lobe defects. *Cortex, 12,* 313–324. (Available from Psychological Assessment Resources, Inc. Odessa, FL).

Van Mourik, M., Verschaeve, P., Boon, P., & Harskamp, F. (1992). Cognition in global aphasia: Indicators for therapy. *Aphasiology, 5,* 491–500.

Vignolo, L. A. (1989). Non-verbal conceptual impairment in aphasia. In F. Boller & J. Grafman (Eds.). *Handbook of Neuropsychology* (Vol. 2, pp. 185–206). New York: Elsevier.

Wechsler, D. (1987). *Wechsler Memory Scale–Revised.* New York: The Psychological Corp.

Wepman, J. (1972). Aphasia therapy. A new look. *Journal of Speech and Hearing Disorders, 37,* 203–214.

CHAPTER

5

An Experimental Treatment of Sentence Comprehension

RITA SLOAN BERNDT, Ph.D.
CHARLOTTE C. MITCHUM, M.S., CCC-SLP

I. BACKGROUND

A. Sentence Comprehension in Aphasia

It is well known that some aphasic patients experience disruption of the ability to understand language; comprehension assessment is routinely included in clinical aphasia batteries (e.g., Goodglass & Kaplan, 1983; Kertesz, 1979). One common form of comprehension impairment that is not routinely tested is uncovered when patients fail to interpret sentences containing two or more nouns that could be the agent of the sentence verb (Berndt & Caramazza, 1980; Saffran & Schwartz, 1988). For example, the ability to recognize that two different sentences can describe the same scene (e.g., "The girl is kicking the boy" and "The boy is kicked by the girl") requires interpretation of both the form of the verb and the order of the nouns around the verb. Patients who are impaired in their ability to interpret these structural cues from sentences may depend on other factors to interpret the sentences they hear (Berndt, Mitchum, & Haendiges, 1996). For example, a patient might assume that the first mentioned noun is always the agent of the action. This strategy would fail for sentences that do not follow agent-first word order, such as those in the passive voice. This type of difficulty understanding reversible sentences is observed in tests that are specifically constructed to assess interpretation of sentence structure. One such test is sentence-picture matching in which the only difference between the target picture and its alternative(s) depends on correct interpretation of which noun is the agent of the action (see Figure 5–1A).

Poor comprehension of semantically reversible sentences is often observed along with *intact* comprehension of "semantically nonreversible" sentences—sentences in which only one of the nouns could logically carry out the sentence action, such as "the ball is kicked by the girl." Superior comprehension of nonreversible sentences in these patients presumably depends on the knowledge that "girls," but not "balls," can "kick" (see Figure 5–1B); interpretation of structure is constrained by meaning. Patients' ability to interpret nonreversible sentences, despite failure to understand reversible sentences, underscores the structural/syntactic nature of their comprehension impairment.

B. Functional Significance

The inability to interpret sentence structure can seriously undermine functional comprehension. The types of sentence structures at risk are very common in conversational interaction. The aspect of language comprehension at issue here is among the most basic: interpreting the sentence cues that indicate WHO is doing what to WHOM. For example, a patient who is unable to distinguish the meaning of "the ball was hit to Ripken" from "the ball was hit by Ripken" might have great difficulty listening to a baseball game on the radio. Clearly, a demonstration of *good* comprehension on clinical batteries does not necessarily mean that the patient consistently performs the essential task of assigning the role of agent to the correct noun. Many patients who are well recovered from other aspects of language impairment, and who are perhaps many years postonset of aphasia, continue to fail to understand the significance of variations in sentence structures. Thus, an important research goal is the development of treatments that can be used to address these frequent residual deficits.

A. Target and distractor stimuli to probe comprehension of sentence meaning ("the girl is kicking the boy") against a semantic reversal foil ("the boy is kicking the girl").

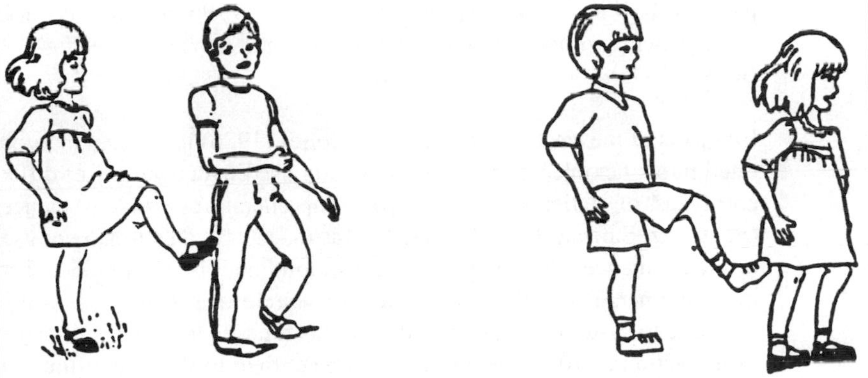

B. Target and verb distractor stimuli to probe comprehension of semantically nonreversible sentence meaning ("the girl is kicking the ball") against a verb meaning foil ("the girl is throwing the ball").

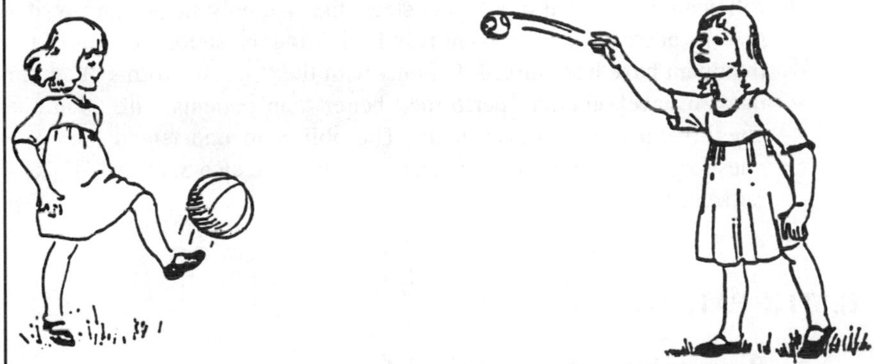

Figure 5–1. Sample items of a sentence-picture matching test designed to assess comprehension of semantically reversible (A) and semantically nonreversible (B) sentences

C. Previous Treatments for Sentence Comprehension Disorder

The earliest discussions of the type of comprehension disorder at issue here focused on the occurrence of the comprehension problem in patients with "agrammatic" speech—those Broca's aphasic patients with significant omissions of grammatical morphemes in their sentence *production.* Early treatments likewise focused on these types of patients (Byng, 1988; Jones, 1986), with emphasis on the relationships among aspects of comprehension and production impairments. It is now clear, however, that this type of comprehension impairment does not always occur when patients show agrammatic speech (Berndt et al., 1996) and does occur in some patients without agrammatic speech (e.g., Mitchum, Haendiges, & Berndt, 1995).

Elements of the treatment designed by Jones (1986) have been incorporated into a flexible treatment program and used with a variety of different types of patients who fail to comprehend reversible sentences (Schwartz, Saffran, Fink, Myers, & Martin, 1994). This treatment uses printed sentences that the patient reads aloud and are then modeled by the examiner. The patient is instructed to circle words in a sentence in response to systematic queries. Attention is focused first to identification of the action (verb) in the printed sentence, then to the role of the sentence nouns in relationship to the action. "WH-questions" are used to guide identification of the noun roles of *agent* ["Which one is doing the (verb)ing?"] versus the *undergoer* of the action ["What is he or she (verb)ing?"]. Immediate feedback is given for each trial by allowing the patient to compare his or her response to a "key." Correct responses are followed by a verbal model that states the written sentence and verifies that the noun selected as agent is indeed doing the action. Results of this treatment have been mixed. Patients with the "purest" forms of agrammatism have generally performed better than patients with additional cognitive/linguistic impairments. The ability to understand the "WH questions" is an important predictive factor (see also Schwartz, Fink, & Saffran, 1995).

II. THE PATIENT

A. Biography and Medical History

FM was a 38-year-old, right-handed, high school educated truck driver in 1981 when he suffered a complete occlusion of the left internal carotid artery. Residual symptoms of the CVA included moderate hemiparesis, mild dysarthria, and moderately severe agrammatic Broca's aphasia. FM experienced an excellent functional recovery and has continued many of his premorbid activities, including boating and other family activities. In 1992, at the time of this study, he regularly drove to the laboratory for his appointments, and he worked part-time in a carryout sandwich shop.

B. Language Status at Treatment Initiation

FM's speech was "agrammatic" as classically defined: halting speech with production of few grammatical function words, main verbs, or bound grammatical markers. FM has participated in many research studies of these features of his agrammatism (Berndt, Haendiges, Mitchum, & Sandson, 1997; Saffran, Berndt, & Schwartz, 1989). His sentence comprehension also has been studied extensively by several different research groups (Badecker, Nathan, & Caramazza, 1991; Berndt, Salasoo, Mitchum, & Blumstein, 1988; Ostrin & Schwartz, 1986). These studies document that comprehension of active- and passive-voice reversible sentences has remained remarkably consistent, yielding chance-level performance for both active and passive sentences in six assessments obtained over a 10-year period.

III. APPRAISAL

A. Rationale

A baseline assessment was designed to allow interpretation of the separate elements that contributed to FM's persistent comprehension impairment and to provide a means of evaluating the precise locus of any changes brought about by the treatment. Five tests were designed to evaluate comprehension of the meanings of isolated verbs, of reversible sentences with locative prepositions, and of reversible declarative sentences under three different conditions.

B. Methods

The five assessments discussed here, along with some additional tests, were presented to FM prior to the introduction of any treatment. None of the tests described below is a published test, nor are they subtests of any standard test battery. Rather, each test was designed to address a specific hypothesis regarding the nature of FM's sentence processing abilities.

1. Comprehension of Verb Meanings

a. **Photo matching.** Thirty picturable verbs were frequency-matched to an equal number of picturable nouns. For each word, a photograph of the target action or object was paired with a distractor photograph of a closely related activity (for verbs) or object (for nouns). FM was asked to point to the one photograph of the pair that best depicted the spoken word (which for verbs used the uninflected form).

b. **Video verb comprehension test.** Ten pairs of videotaped action scenes were presented in split-screen format. The word pairs were related in meaning (e.g., hit/kick; hug/kiss); both verbs of each pair were tested, for a total of 20 trials. After the examiner read the target, each scene was presented individually on half of the video screen. FM responded by pointing to one of the depictions on the screen.

2. Comprehension of Reversible Sentences

a. **Locative prepositions.** Eight locative prepositions were used to construct a sentence/picture matching task that probed interpretation of preposition meaning (e.g., "The shoe is *in* the box" versus "The shoe is *on* the box") and, importantly, appreciation of noun order (e.g., "The *shoe* is in the *box*" versus "The *box* is in the *shoe*"). Line drawings were constructed to illustrate each target and distractor item. Each preposition was presented as a target in 10 trials that contrasted the target depiction with one distractor; pictures were arrayed vertically. FM was instructed to point to the most appropriate depiction on hearing the spoken target sentence. The full set of trials was administered in 4 blocks of 40 items each.

b. **Standard reversible and nonreversible sentences.** Twenty-four sentences in the active or passive voice were randomly presented, each with a picture pair from which the patient was to choose the one described by the sentence. Half the sentences were semantically reversible (e.g., "The girl is kicking the boy") and half were nonreversible (e.g., "The girl is kicking the ball"). Pictures for the reversible sentences included a depiction of the target and a "reversed role" distractor (boy kicking girl). Distractor pictures for nonreversible sentences employed semantically related lexical contrasts (girl *throwing* ball, see Figure 5–1). Target sentences were arranged in 4 blocks to assure that the same picture pair appeared only once in a block.

c. **Truncated reversible sentences.** The 12 reversible sentences from **2.b.** were modified by deleting the second noun phrase and were administered with the same pair of pictures in active and in passive form. For example, "The boy is kicking the

Table 5-1. Proportion correct responses, baseline assessment obtained with FM

Verb comprehension	
Photo-matching (N = 30)	0.93
Video-matching (N = 20)	1.00
Locative sentence comprehension	
Lexical distractors (N = 80)	0.96
Reversal distractors (N = 80)	0.94
Standard, active/passive voice	
Non-reversible (N = 12)	1.00/0.92
Reversible (N = 12)	0.58/0.58
Truncated, active/passive	
Reversible (N = 12)	0.67/0.67
Agent identification, active/passive	
Reversible (N = 12)	1.00/0.08

girl," was spoken as, "The boy is kicking"; "The boy is kicked by the girl," was presented as, "The boy is kicked." This task explores the importance of the "by" phrase as a signal of a passive voice sentence. Task requirements were otherwise the same as for **2.b.**

d. **Agent identification task.** The semantically reversible sentences from **2.b.** were again administered, but with a different set of picture choices. In this variant, the nouns named in the sentence were pictured in isolation, unengaged in any activity. Thus, "The boy is kicking the girl," was spoken while a picture of a boy and a picture of a girl were presented. FM was instructed to "point to the one who is kicking." This task probed any contribution to the comprehension impairment of difficulties in interpreting actions from static depictions.

C. Results of Baseline Assessment

As shown in Table 5–1, FM demonstrated excellent comprehension of the meanings of isolated verbs, of reversible sentences with locative prepositions, and of nonreversible sentences. In contrast, he displayed marked difficulty with all of the variants of active and passive reversible sentences that were administered.

IV. DIAGNOSIS

A. Interpretation of the Underlying Disorder

The results in Table 5–1 suggest that FM's sentence comprehension failure was not caused by an inability to understand verb meanings. He was clearly able to distinguish between verbs that are closely related semantically. Nor does his sentence comprehension failure seem to have been based on a general inability to interpret word order—he easily understood reversible locative sentences. This result stands in contrast to the general finding that failure to comprehend reversible sentences is typically found in sentences with prepositions as well as in sentences with verbs (Schwartz, Saffran, & Marin, 1980). It would appear from this baseline assessment that FM's difficulty was related to interpreting aspects of sentence structure other than word order.

B. Other Considerations

Although FM has consistently displayed equally poor performance with active and passive voice, a strong bias to the active interpretation emerged in the testing condition in which the actors and action were not fully depicted (agent identification). We interpret this finding as an indication that results of "good" performance with actives should be interpreted with caution—strategies of assigning the agent role to the first noun of the sentence are frequently adopted in unusual testing situations. FM had been tested on the standard sentence-picture-matching (forced-choice) test many times, and it is possible that he had developed strategies and heuristics for its execution that we had not anticipated. His responses to treatment will therefore need to be carefully analyzed for evidence of fluctuating strategies.

V. PROGNOSIS

A. Prognostic Signs

Little is known about the prognosis for sentence comprehension therapies. Nevertheless, good comprehension of nonreversible and locative sentences, along with relatively intact single word comprehension, indicated that FM was an excellent candidate for treatment to improve reversible sentence comprehension. The lengthy time postonset might be a negative prognostic sign, if it indicates that he must "unlearn" some unsuccessful adaptive strategies that interfere with accurate interpretation of reversible sentences.

B. Expected Outcome

As the focus of treatment is strictly within the bounds of sentence processing, generalization of successful reversible sentence interpretation beyond the sentence level is welcomed, but is not necessarily expected. Comprehension at the conversational level may introduce complexities that are not addressed in this narrowly defined intervention.

VI. FOCUSING THE TREATMENT

A. Rationale

In light of FM's good appreciation of word order in the locative sentence comprehension task, it was likely that his impairment with active and passive sentences involved the grammatical function words and bound morphemes that distinguish active from passive voice. It seemed advisable, therefore, that the treatment activities not *require* understanding of the "wh" question words that have been used in treatment of this disorder (Schwartz et al., 1994). Instead, we used a treatment that relied only on feedback to the patient regarding whether or not his responses were correct (Figure 5–2). The training aspect of the procedure consisted of systematic and immediate feedback in which the patient was told whether or not a response was correct. In addition to alerting the patient as to his or her performance, the feedback procedure also illustrated *how* the correct picture corresponded to the components of the spoken sentence (for details see Haendiges, Berndt, & Mitchum, 1996; Mitchum et al., 1995). Treatments based on such "passive" feedback could provide a general approach to the treatment of disorders among "high level" patients who bring an analytic and thoughtful approach to the treatment session.

B. Methods

The feedback approach to treatment of sentence comprehension was adopted in two different sentence-picture-matching situations. At Level 1, one picture and one sentence were presented, and the patient was asked to say whether or not the sentence was an adequate description of the picture. At Level 2, two pictures were presented with a single spoken sentence, and the patient was to choose the picture that best represented the sentence. This paradigm is comparable to the technique used in the baseline assessment.

    1. Materials. Ten transitive verbs not used in the baseline assessment were combined in sentences with two nouns to yield a set of seman-

Scenario: WOMAN SPLASHING MAN

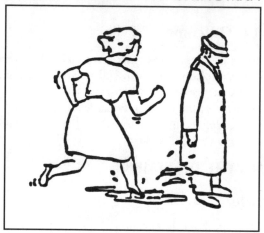

FEEDBACK TO CORRECT RESPONSES

(Stimulus)	(Target)	(Response)	(Feedback)
(Active Sentences)			
"The woman is splashing the man."	Yes	"Yes"	"That's right. . . The woman is splashing the man."
"The man is splashing the woman."	No	"No"	"Right, it's the other way. . . The woman is splashing the man."
(Passive Sentences)			
"The man is splashed by the woman."	Yes	"Yes"	"That's right. . . The man is splashed by the woman."
"The woman is splashed by the man."	No	"No"	"Right, it's the other way. . . The man is splashed by the woman."

FEEDBACK TO INCORRECT RESPONSES

(Stimulus)	(Target)	(Response)	(Feedback)
(Active Sentences)			
"The woman is splashing the man."	Yes	"No"	"It's yes. . . The woman is splashing the man."
"The man is splashing the woman."	No	"Yes"	"No, it was wrong. . . The woman is splashing the man."
(Passive Sentences)			
"The man is splashed by the woman."	Yes	"No"	"It's yes. . . The man is splashed by the woman."
"The woman is splashed by the man."	No	"Yes"	"No, it was wrong. . . The man is splashed by the woman."

Figure 5–2. Sample stimulus for training interpretation of semantically reversible sentences in the "Yes/No" picture-sentence matching paradigm

tically reversible scenarios. Each scenario was drawn once with the agent shown on the right and once with the agent on the left. The same left/right control of agent position was carried out for the reversed scenario. These controls were introduced to prevent the use of spatial strategies from systematically affecting the data (Deloche & Seron, 1981). Thus, four pictures were constructed for each of the 10 verbs. These were used as the picture choices to test comprehension of both active and passive sentences.

2. **Therapeutic Procedures.** The same structure was used in each feedback session to control inadvertent cues and examiner reactions. Spoken practice by FM was inhibited to prevent him from generating conflicting auditory/verbal information. As noted, two types of interaction used the same pictures, but provided a slightly different method of feedback.

   a. **Yes/no, one picture.** This condition controlled the presentation of stimuli to equate the number of active and passive sentences, the number of times each noun was depicted as the agent of the action, the right/left position of the agent in the picture and the number of matched/mismatched trials. These controls yielded a total of 16 trials per verb for each of 10 verbs. One picture was shown to FM as a sentence was spoken aloud. All sentences contained lexical items that matched the picture, but in half the trials the sentence meaning represented a reversal of the depiction. FM was instructed to say "yes" if the sentence described the picture and "no" if it did not. FM was told immediately whether or not his response was correct. If correct, the sentence was repeated for him; if incorrect, the sentence was spoken in the same (active/passive) voice with nouns rearranged to be in the correct order, while he continued to study the picture.

   b. **Forced choice, two pictures.** At Level 2, FM was shown two alternative depictions of the same actors engaged in an action. One of the pictures matched the spoken sentence, and the other showed a reversal of the noun roles. The pictures were arranged vertically for presentation, with the target appearing equally on top or bottom.

3. **General Procedures.** Seven full administrations (i.e., "rounds") of 160 trials of yes/no matching were preceded by 2 pretraining rounds with no feedback. Prior to providing any feedback, one assessment without feedback was administered for the forced choice

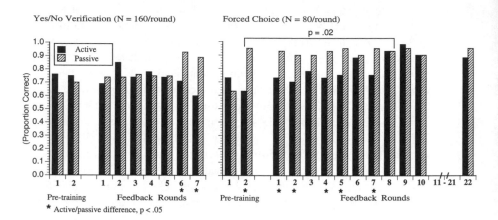

Figure 5–3. Proportion correct performance by FM on reversible active and passive voice sentences in each complete administration ("round") of the training materials

procedure as well. A second assessment in the forced choice condition was obtained on completion of the yes/no training, but prior to the start of the forced choice training trial.

C. Results

FM's responses during the therapy were analyzed in terms of the overall proportion of correct responses obtained in each complete "round" with feedback relative to the proportion of correct responses obtained with no feedback (pretraining), and with regard to active/passive performance differences. Figure 5–3 displays FM's performance for each round.

1. **Overall Proportion Correct.** In the "yes/no" condition, the overall proportion of correct responses did not increase appreciably between the pretraining assessments (0.69 and 0.73 correct) and the final (seventh) round of treatment (0.74 correct). Similarly, there was no significant change in proportion of correct responses observed between the first (0.68 correct) and second (0.79 correct) forced choice pretests ($\chi^2 = 2.04$, $p = 0.15$), despite the 7 rounds of "yes/no" feedback that occurred between them. However, in the 8th full round of the forced choice procedure with feedback, a significant increase in total number of correct responses was observed (from 0.79 correct in pretest 2 to 0.93 correct at round 8; $\chi^2 = 5.08$, $p = 0.02$). An additional series of rounds was administered in an attempt to establish perfect performance. Although accuracy

failed to reach 100% after 22 full rounds, a consistent range of 0.91 to 0.95 correct was maintained.

2. **Performance Pattern.** A significant difference in performance with active and passive targets was noted at several points during the feedback trials. As shown in Figure 5–3, initially a somewhat larger proportion of active targets was correct (pretraining 1 of the yes/no condition, active/passive difference $\chi^2 = 3.14$, $p = 0.08$). A shift in the pattern in favor of passive targets emerged at round 6 of the yes/no condition and was maintained in the (second) pretraining assessment and several early rounds of the forced choice procedure (i.e., 5 of the first 7 rounds). Later rounds of forced choice were quite accurate in response to both active and passive targets. This gradual shift from more correct responses with active, then with passive, and finally to consistently correct performance on both sentence types, suggests that FM's change in interpretation of the reversible sentences involved some shift in response strategy as he attempted to align elements of sentences with their pictured representations. The appreciation of structural cues unique to each sentence type apparently evolved for FM over the course of many trials with immediate feedback regarding the correctness of his response.

3. **Generalization to Untrained Materials.** To assess the generality of FM's improved comprehension of the treatment sentences, the three sets of baseline tests on which he had performed poorly were readministered. To assure the stability of the data in the two conditions in which the outcome was not definitive on the first posttreatment assessment (truncated and agent identification tasks), a second assessment was obtained for those tasks. This posttreatment testing was carried out in conjunction with the administration of other tasks in weekly sessions over 6 weeks.

Figure 5–4 presents a comparison of the baseline and posttraining assessments, collapsing across sentence voice to look at overall proportion correct. Although there was some improvement over baseline in all posttraining assessments, this change was significant only for the standard testing format (McNemar test, B(aseline) 1 versus P(ost) = 2.83, $p = 0.002$; B2 versus P = 2.11, $p = 0.02$) and the agent identification task (B1 versus P1, B2 versus P2, McNemar test = 2.36, $p = 0.01$). The two tasks that improved employed the active and passive sentence structures that had been trained but contained new lexical content. The task that did not show significant improvement used truncated sentences, which have a syntactic structure that differs from the training stimuli. Thus, although the

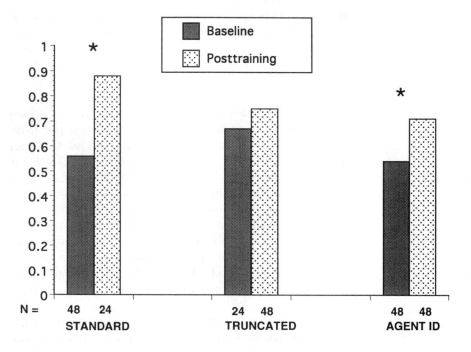

*McNemar Test (one-tailed), baseline and posttraining, p>.01

Figure 5–4. Overall proportion correct performance (collapsed across active/passive) on untrained reversible sentences by patient FM in three tasks administered at baseline and following training

therapeutic procedure effectively generalized to interpretation of active and passive sentences with untrained *lexical* content, it would appear that these results were contingent on processing the fully expressed sentence structure that had been used in training.

4. **Item Analysis on Individual Sentences.** Despite the generalization of the training effects to untrained materials, several aspects of the training and assessment data suggest that the effectiveness of the feedback procedure might have been at least partly influenced by differences in sentence meaning. First, the prefeedback assessments with the training materials (see pretraining data in Figure 5–3) yielded consistently better performance (70% and above) than did the baseline assessments with the same (i.e., standard) testing format but different lexical content (less than 60% correct). Second, despite significant and consistent improvement in the later feedback

rounds, FM's performance levels with the training materials never reached ceiling. An item analysis was carried out on the sentences used in the training in an attempt to determine if these unexplained aspects of the data were related to differential performance on specific sentences.

Training rounds 8–22 showed a level of performance significantly improved over the pretraining assessments. These were used to determine if there were differences among specific sentences even after performance approached ceiling. Sentences using 6 of the 10 training verbs resulted in a mean performance level in rounds 8–22 of 95% correct or better, with equivalent performance on active and passive sentences ($N = 120$/verb). FM was able to interpret both active and passive voice structures in sentences using these verbs. Sentences containing the remaining 4 training verbs never reached a consistently high level of performance, even after many rounds of feedback and despite excellent performance with sentences using other verbs. For one of these verbs ("bite"), the problem appeared to involve sentence plausibility rather than structural factors. Pictures used with this verb contrasted the scenarios "dog bites man" with "man bites dog," the latter depicted by a cartoon-like figure on hands and knees biting a dog on the tail. In the forced choice trials using "bite" in rounds 8–22 ($N = 120$), FM was correct significantly more often on the active and passive sentences in which the correct interpretation was "dog bites man" (92%) than on sentences in which the correct interpretation was "man bites dog" (67% correct; $\chi^2 = 9.90$, $p = 0.002$) Despite the ability of control subjects and at least one other aphasic patient (see Mitchum et al., 1995) to accommodate the somewhat unlikely (but possible) scenario of a man biting a dog, FM was apparently very unwilling to violate his expectation about which picture was most likely to occur in the real world. Unlike "bite," 3 other verbs that failed to reach ceiling levels in the training seemed to be understood in ways that consistently favored either an active or a passive interpretation.

An item analysis was also carried out on the assessment materials, using the "standard" and agent identification tasks that showed improvement following the feedback rounds. The number of trials for sentences using each of the 6 verbs included in this set of materials was considerably smaller than for the training materials: the baseline included two complete administrations of each of the two tasks, for a total of 8 trials per verb for each sentence type; the posttest included a single administration of the standard task and two administrations of the agent identification task, for a total of

Table 5–2. Summary of FM's sentence comprehension performance for each verb in late stages of training and posttraining assessment

	"Good" Verbs	**"Poor" Verbs**
Training Set	(95%, A = P)	(75–92% with significant A–P difference)
(Rounds 8–22, $n = 120$)	wash splash find hold shoot	bite tow pay carry
Assessment Set	(significant change from baseline)	(no significant change from baseline)
(Posttraining assessment standard sentences and agent ID, $n = 6$)	push hit pull	follow scare chase

6 trials/verb for each sentence type. Overall performance at baseline for sentences using each verb ranged from 0.50 to 0.69 correct; no verb was associated with performance at above chance levels (all $p > 0.10$, binomial test).

Sentences using 3 of the 6 assessment verbs were comprehended significantly better following the training: sentences using "push" changed from 0.63 to 0.92 correct (FI = 2.93, $p = .04$); sentences using "hit" changed from 0.56 to 0.92 (FI = 4.07, $p = 0.02$); and sentences with "pull" changed from 0.50 to 0.83 (FI = 3.18, $p = 0.03$). Sentences with the remaining 3 verbs ("follow," "scare," and "chase") showed some improvement, but the change was not reliable. Moreover, sentences with "follow" continued to show a major effect of sentence voice at the posttest, with consistent choices of the correct picture for active sentences and of the incorrect picture for passive sentences. Table 5–2 summarizes these distinctions between the verbs that were ultimately "good" and those that remained "poor" for the training and the assessment verb sets.

The appearance of these verb-specific effects in FM's sentence comprehension performance after successful treatment is unlikely to indicate a basic impairment of verb comprehension. Baseline testing had demonstrated excellent comprehension of nuances of verb meaning. Rather, some interaction of verb meaning with inter-

pretation of sentence structure must underlie this continued difficulty with some verbs.

VII. DISCUSSION

A. Rationale: Locus of Treatment Effects

The treatment to improve FM's comprehension did not provide explicit
instruction about which sentence elements were important for mapping
or what they signified. Rather, the "training" repeatedly paired sentence
structure with meaning, and it was left to FM to infer that the two syntactic structures had different consequences for interpretation. At the end of
training, his ability to identify the agent noun was much improved for
both sentence types, demonstrating that the treatment effectively produced the intended result. This new-found ability was not specific to the
lexical content of the training stimuli, as shown by generalization to
untrained sentences. It was, however, limited to the sentence structures
used in the training procedure, as indicated by the lack of generalization
to comprehension of truncated structures. Comprehension of truncated
sentences is necessarily based on interpretation of elements of verb morphology; fully expressed sentences contain an additional cue to sentence
voice in the presence of the "by phrase" containing the agent noun. The
success of this treatment, although clearly circumscribed in its generalization, is an important demonstration of significant improvement in the
ability of a chronic aphasic patient to work out relationships between
structural sentence elements and meaning. The changes established in
sentence interpretation were clearly a demonstration of the therapeutic
effects of consistent feedback about which interpretations were correct.

B. Hindsight: Control of Verb Meanings

Most importantly, FM's ability to interpret sentences at the end of training was clearly affected by the verbs used in the sentences. As in most
studies of this issue, verbs were not selected to have any particular syntactic or semantic characteristics other than picturability and the ability
to be used plausibly in a reversible sentence. Post hoc attempts to determine why FM's comprehension at the end of training was so much better
for some verbs than for others uncovered no obvious structural differences (e.g., Grimshaw, 1990) between the easy and difficult verbs. In
addition, factors that have previously been invoked (Jones, 1984; Saffran, Schwartz, & Marin, 1980) failed to predict the hierarchy of difficulty found here.

A new approach to the question of why a patient might experience different degrees of difficulty when assigning thematic roles to different

verbs adopts a modified view of the relation between verb representations and thematic roles. In contrast to the traditional position that each predicate assigns a discrete thematic role (agent, theme, etc.) from a list of possible roles to each of its arguments (Jackendoff, 1972), Dowty (1991) has proposed that verbs assign arguments to one of two cluster-concepts (proto-agent or proto-patient) through a set of verbal entailments. An argument of a verb may bear either of the proto-roles (or both) to varying degrees, depending on the number of entailments of each kind that is carried by the verb. Verb entailments for the proto-agent role include factors such as volitional involvement in the event, sentience or perception of the event, causality of the event or of a change of state in another participant, movement relative to another participant, and existence independent of the event. Entailments for the proto-patient role include complementary characteristics, such as undergoing a change of state. For present purposes, the importance of this formulation is that verbs may differ in the number of entailments falling into each of these concept clusters, resulting in more or less clear assignment of arguments to (deep) subject and object.

If these notions are applied to the data from FM, there is some reason to view the "difficult" verbs as less clearly agentive than are the "easy" verbs; that is, there were differences among the verbs in entailments such as relative motion, volition, and causality. The verbs that FM learned to interpret in reversible sentences clearly entail properties that strongly constrain identification of the agent noun. As interpreted in the pictures used to test comprehension, each of them involved notable asymmetries of movement between the two participants (with the patient essentially motionless as in "splash"), and/or a marked change of state being brought about in one of the participants (e.g., "shoot"). This notion of asymmetry of movement/change of state also helps to draw a distinction among the directional verbs FM found to be "easy" ("push," "pull," where the patient is passive and stationary) and those he treated as more "difficult" ("follow," "chase," where agent and patient are equally active and moving). The verbs that were not interpreted correctly at the end of training involved much more symmetrical levels of motion between the participants and little evidence of any change of state in the noun filling the thematic role of patient.

The proposal here is that, despite generally good comprehension of verb meanings demonstrated in single word tasks, FM was unable to assign "agent" status to arguments for verbs without clear verb entailments indicating agency. The precise source of this problem—whether it involves verb comprehension alone or in interaction with picture interpretation—is still unclear. Research is continuing on this question.

VIII. CONCLUSION

Among the many issues raised by the results of this study, two have particularly important clinical relevance. First, analysis of the item-specific treatment effects obtained with FM demonstrates that the selection of training and assessment materials must be carried out with careful attention to the nature of the stimuli in the context of the task demands. A verb-sensitive pattern of performance was not evident until the treatment results were analyzed, and performance for some sentences improved beyond what would be expected by chance. Studies of treatment effects that look for generalization to new materials must be based on the assumption that the untreated materials are comparable to the treatment materials in every way *except* that they are "new" to the patient. This study has shown that structurally comparable sentences may not be identical in terms of the important information that a patient may need to use in the task at hand. It is difficult to predict the factors that will be most important in determining comparability across materials, but research is continuing on identifying such factors.

Second, this study is part of a continuing effort to demonstrate the benefits that focused treatment can have on the residual language disabilities of chronic aphasic patients (see, for example, papers in Berndt & Mitchum, 1995). Although practical constraints on the delivery of services may prevent widespread intervention with such patients, it is clear that effective, well-targeted intervention can bring about change even after many years of chronic language disorder. For experimental demonstration, it is often necessary to study specific treatment effects in patients for whom the language impairment is static; interpretation of treatment effects is difficult enough without the necessity of measuring spontaneous recovery. The question remains, however, whether the treatment described here would have a similar beneficial effect on the sentence comprehension impairment of patients with more dynamic (perhaps acute) language impairment or even if such focused treatment would be possible in the acute stage. The general applicability of this approach requires further testing. Nevertheless, this form of treatment efficacy research provides a clear demonstration of the important relationship between clinical intervention and theoretical interpretation of the cognitive disorder that underlies aphasic language.

IX. ACKNOWLEDGMENTS

This project was supported by Grant Number R01-DC00262 from the National Institutes of Health. The authors are grateful to Anne N. Haendiges for help in planning treatment, to Lisa Bayne for assistance with data management, and to Sarah C. Wayland for assistance with the verb analysis. The dedicated participation of patient FM in this research is also gratefully acknowledged.

X. REFERENCES

Badecker, W., Nathan, P., & Carmazza, A. (1991). Varieties of sentence comprehension deficits. A case study. *Cortex 27*, 31–321.

Berndt, R. S., & Caramazza, A. (1980). A redefinition of the syndrome of Broca's aphasia: Implications for a neuropsychological model of language. *Applied Psycholinguistics 1*, 225–278.

Berndt, R. S., Haendiges, A. N., Mitchum, C. C., & Sandson, J. (1997). Verb retrieval in aphasia: 2. Relationship to sentence processing. *Brain and Language, 56*, 107–137.

Berndt, R. S., & Mitchum, C. C. (1995). *Cognitive neuropsychological approaches to the treatment of language disorders.* Hove, UK: Lawrence Erlbaum Associates.

Berndt, R. S., Mitchum, C. C., & Haendiges, A. N. (1996). Comprehension of reversible sentences in "agrammatism": A meta-analysis. *Cognition 58*, 289–308.

Berndt, R. S., Salasoo, A., Mitchum, C. C., & Blumstein, S. E. (1988). The role of intonation cues in aphasic patients' performance of the grammaticality judgment task. *Brain and Language, 34*, 65–97.

Byng, S. (1988). Sentence processing deficits: Theory and therapy. *Cognitive Neuropsychology, 5*, 629–676.

Deloche, G., & Seron, X. (1981). Sentence understanding and knowledge of the world: Evidence from a sentence-picture matching task performed by aphasic patients. *Brain and Language 14*, 57–69.

Dowty, D. (1991). Thematic proto-roles and argument selection. *Language 67*, 547–619.

Goodglass, H., & Kaplan, E. (1983). *Boston Diagnostic Aphasic Examination* (2nd ed.). Philadelphia: Lea & Febiger.

Grimshaw, J. (1990). *Argument structure.* Cambridge: MIT Press.

Haendiges, A. N., Berndt, R. S., & Mitchum, C. C. (1996). Assessing the elements contributing to a "mapping" deficit: A targeted treatment study. *Brain and Language 52*, 276–302.

Jackendoff, R. (1972). *Semantic interpretation of generative grammar.* Cambridge: MIT Press.

Jones, E. V. (1984). Word order processing in aphasia: Effect of verb semantics. In F. C. Rose (Ed.), *Advances in neurology: Progress in aphasiology* (pp. 159–181). New York: Raven Press.

Jones, E. V. (1986). Building the foundations for sentence production in a non-fluent aphasic. *British Journal of Disorders of Communications, 21*(1), 63–82.

Kertesz, A. (1979). *Aphasia and associated disorders: Taxonomy, localization, and recovery.* New York: Grune & Stratton.

Mitchum, C. C., Haendiges, A. N., & Berndt, R. S. (1995). Treatment of thematic mapping in sentence comprehension: Implications for normal processing. *Cognitive Neuropsychology, 12*, 503–547.

Ostrin, R. K., & Schwartz, M. F. (1986). Reconstructing from a degraded trace: A study of sentence repetition in agrammatism. *Brain and Language, 28*, 328–345.

Saffran, E. M., Berndt, R. S., & Schwartz, M. F. (1989). The quantitative analysis of agrammatic production: Procedure and data. *Brain and Language 37*, 440–479.

Saffran, E. M., & Schwartz, M. F. (1988). 'Agrammatic' comprehension it's not: Alternative and implications. *Aphasiology, 2*, 389–394.

Saffran, E. M., Schwartz, M. F., & Marin, O. S. M. (1980). The word order problem in agrammatism: Production. *Brain and Language, 10*, 263–280.

Schwartz, M. F., Fink, R. B., & Saffran, E. M. (1995). The modular treatment of agrammatism. *Neuropsychological rehabilitation 5*(1/2), 93–127.

Schwartz, M. F., Saffran, E. M., Fink, R. B., Myers, J., & Martin, N. (1994). Mapping therapy: A treatment programme for agrammatism. *Aphasiology 8*, 19–54.

Schwartz, M. F., Saffran, E. M., & Marin, O. S. M. (1980). The word order problem in agrammatism: Comprehension. *Brain and Language, 10*, 249–262.

CHAPTER

6

Treating Sentence Production in Agrammatic Aphasia

CYNTHIA K. THOMPSON, PH.D.

This chapter describes the treatment provided for a patient with agrammatic aphasia. When first evaluated the patient, JD, was 44 years old and 2 years post stroke. Although his aphasia had improved markedly in the first 2 years, his language remained impaired. His reading and auditory comprehension were fairly well preserved, but his sentence production, both in writing and in speaking, was agrammatic.

Before the treatment provided for JD is discussed, some of the key characteristics of agrammatic aphasia and theoretical accounts of agrammatism are presented. Then JD's medical history, tests administered, and test results are presented. A description of the treatments provided over a 1½-year-period, the rationale for selecting these treatments, and how they affected JD's aphasia are then discussed.

In the final section, alternative treatment possibilities and JD's continuing treatment needs are addressed.

I. BACKGROUND

A. The Nature of Agrammatic Aphasia

1. The Language Deficit. Agrammatic aphasia is typically seen in individuals with nonfluent Broca's aphasia. The disorder refers to a pattern of sentence production that reflects an absence of grammatical structure while comprehension remains relatively spared (Goodglass, 1976; also see deBlesser, 1987 for historical review). Individuals with agrammatism speak effortfully, frequently omitting grammatical function words and inflections, but often convey adequate messages by using structurally impoverished strings of content words. A number of detailed accounts of agrammatic language patterns have been advanced in recent research. Results of this research have shown the following characteristics:

a. Difficulty with production of bound and/or free standing grammatical morphemes (see for example Caramazza & Hillis, 1989; Micelli, Silveri, Romani, & Caramazza, 1989).

b. Production of more open-class than closed-class words (see for example Menn, 1990; Miceli, Silveri, Villa, & Caramazza, 1984).

c. Difficulty with production of verbs and an overreliance on nouns (Kohn, Lorch, & Pearson, 1989; Miceli et al., 1984; Miceli, Silveri, & Nocentini, & Caramazza, 1988; Zingeser & Berndt, 1990).

d. Production of simple verbs with simple argument structure[1] and impoverished production of adjuncts[2] (Caplan & Hanna, in press; Thompson, Lange, Schneider, & Shapiro, in press; Thompson, Shapiro, Li, & Schendel, 1995; Thompson, Shapiro, Tait et al., 1995).

---

[1]The number of participants that go into the "action" described by the verb are called arguments of the verb. Arguments are part of the verb's lexical representation.

[2]Adjuncts are phrases contained within sentences that are not a part of a verb's lexical representation; thus they are not obligatory in sentences and they are not assigned a thematic role by a verb. Consider the following sentence: [Zack AGENT] fixed [the toy THEME] [in the closet LOCATION]. The two-place transitive verb *fix* assigns only two thematic roles—Agent to the NP *Zack*, and theme to *the toy*. The PP *in the closet* is a locative adjunct; its "meaning" is not inherent in the verb's representation.

e. Production of short, grammatically ill-formed, syntactically simple utterances (Goodglass, Christiansen, & Gallagher, 1993; Saffran, Berndt, & Schwartz, 1989; Thompson, Shapiro, Tait et al., 1995), and an overuse of elliptical forms (Heeschen, 1985).

f. Difficulty producing complex sentences in which noun phrases (NPs) have been moved out of their subject-verb-object order (Saffran et al., 1989; Thompson, Shapiro, Tait, et al., 1995).

g. Difficulty comprehending noncanonical, semantically reversible sentences, those with complex verbs, or those with more than one verb (see, for example, Caplan, Baker, & Dehaut, 1985; Saffran, Schwartz, & Marin, 1980).

h. Preserved ability to make grammaticality judgments (Linebarger, Schwartz, & Saffran, 1983).

Notably, there is heterogeneity among these characteristics in individual patients and dissociations among the primary characteristics of agrammatism have been reported. Three types of grammatical disturbances were described some years ago by Tissot, Maunin, and Lhermitte (1973), including (a) fragmented, halting, and limited speech output without major structural errors, (b) a primarily morphological impairment in which bound and free-standing grammatical morphemes are missing but word order is intact, and (c) a primarily constructional impairment in which complete sentences are rarely produced, but grammatical morphemes are not impaired. More recent literature has further detailed patterns of impairment in agrammatic patients. For example, patients have shown differential deficits in bound, but not free-standing morphemes (Miceli & Mazzuchi, 1990; Saffran et al., 1989) and within these classes some elements and not others have been affected (Nespoulous et al., 1988; Miceli et al., 1989). Some patients show problems affecting only grammatical morphemes, but not sentence structure per se and vice versa (Berndt, 1987; Saffran et al., 1980). Finally, some (but not all) agrammatic patients present patterns of asyntactic comprehension in which complex, noncanonical sentences, such as passives, are poorly comprehended, but little difficulty is noted with active sentences (Berndt, Mitchum, & Haendiges, 1996; Caplan et al., 1985; Grodzinsky, 1986; Nespoulous et al., 1988). Notably, these patients often show particular difficulty with semantically reversible sentences (i.e., those in which two nouns are equally probable candidates for the thematic role of "Agent").

2. **Theories of Agrammatism.** Many theoretical accounts have been offered to accommodate the performance patterns seen in agrammatism, including linguistic explanations that place the impairment within specific aspects of the syntactic representation that patients can generate (Grodzinsky, 1986, 1995; Mauner, Fromkin, & Cornell, 1993). Other explanations locate the impairment in operations that "map" syntactic roles of nouns to thematic (semantic) roles such as "Agent of the action" (Schwartz, Linebarger, Saffran, & Pate, 1987). Still other theories have suggested that error patterns seen in agrammatism reflect an adaptation to short-term memory limitations, changes in the thresholds of word activation, or an increase in noise in the system (Kolk, Van Grusven, & Keyser, 1985).

Models of normal sentence production also have been used to determine where in the process of sentence planning breakdowns occur in agrammatic aphasia (Bock, 1987; Garrett, 1980, 1984). Garrett's model, for example, includes several stages of sentence planning, from an early conceptual, or inferential, stage where the ideas to be expressed in a sentence are generated to an articulatory stage where the motor codes for production of the sentence are accessed. Using this model, agrammatism has been cast as a disorder resulting from disruption of one of two possible stages of sentence planning: (1) the "functional" level of processing, where open-class words including verbs and their arguments are accessed and thematic roles are assigned (Thompson, Shapiro, & Roberts, 1993), and (2) the "positional" level, a stage where bound and free-standing morphemes are accessed and placed in sentence frames together with content words and the phonology of these elements is specified (Caramazza & Hillis, 1989; Mitchum, 1992). The exact locus of the deficit, however, remains under debate. Clearly, given the different patterns of impairment seen in individuals with agrammatism, it is likely that different aspects of sentence planning may be involved in different patients.

II. THE PATIENT

A. Biography

JD was 44 years old and 2 years post stroke when he was first evaluated in the aphasia research laboratory at Northwestern University. A native

English speaker, he was left-handed and had more than 20 years of formal education. Prior to his stoke he had held a management position in a major corporation. He was married, with two children.

B. Medical History

JD suffered a left hemisphere, cerebral vascular accident (stroke) in the distribution of the middle cerebral artery (MCA). Computerized tomography (CT) scan at 1 month post stroke showed a lesion occupying the frontal operculum and extending to the underlying white matter, the motor cortex, the insula, and the basal ganglia. He had a history of heart disease; thus, the stroke was considered a probable cardiogenic embolus. JD had no history of neurological disease, psychiatric disorders, alcoholism, developmental speech-language disorders, or learning disabilities.

The stroke left him with a right hemiparesis and Broca's aphasia. Production in both speech and writing was reduced to single words, both reading and auditory comprehension were relatively spared, although he showed difficulty understanding numbers, proper names, complex directions, and prepositions.

Immediately following the stroke JD received intensive physical and speech-language therapy. Apparently, his hemiparesis resolved somewhat; when I met him he walked with a cane and brace on the right leg and had no use of his right arm. His aphasia had also improved; after 2 years of speech and language therapy, he was able to produce phrases and occasional sentences, but his writing remained at the single-word level. His comprehension continued to be compromised, but only for complex commands and sentences, and he was able to read 4–5 pages per hour of popular novels, although he reported some difficulty reading prepositions and complex sentences. His hearing was within normal limits.

III. APPRAISAL OF THE APHASIA

A. Testing for Agrammatism

Review of materials provided by JD's speech-language pathologist led us to suspect that he had an agrammatic aphasia. Therefore, a number of tests—both published and unpublished—were administered to examine aspects of language known to be involved in agrammatism. Although standardized aphasia test batteries are inadequate for examining grammatical deficits, they were used as a starting point and followed by further in-depth testing.

Table 6–1. Types of verbs and their argument structure arrangements

Verb type	Sample verb	Argument structure	Sample sentence
One-place	sleep	Agent	(Zack) slept.
Two-place	fix	Agent, Theme	(Zack) fixed (the car).
Three-place (nonalternating)	put	Agent, Theme, Location	(Zack) put (the toy) (in the closet).
Three-Place (alternating)	give	Agent, Theme, Goal	(Zack) gave (the book) (to Tim).
		Agent, Goal, Theme	(Zack) gave (Tim) (the book).
Complement	know	Agent, Theme	(Zack) knew (the answer). (Zack) knew (that Bria left).

B. Method and Results

1. **General Aphasia Testing.** Two aphasia test batteries were administered: The *Porch Index of Communicative Abilities* (PICA, Porch, 1973) and the *Western Aphasia Battery* (WAB, Kertesz, 1982). On the PICA, JD's performance on verbal subtests was worse than on gestural or graphic ones. Results revealed the following percentiles: verbal, 59; gestural, 71; graphic 77; and overall, 72. Similar performance patterns were noted on the WAB. His aphasia quotient (AQ) was 62; his fluency score was 4.0; comprehension, repetition, naming, and reading ranged from 5.0–8.0.

2. **Sentence Comprehension Testing.** Because comprehension of complex sentences often is compromised in individuals with agrammatism, testing was undertaken to examine JD's comprehension ability. Two unpublished measures were selected: The *Philadelphia Comprehension Battery for Aphasia* (PCBA, Saffran, Schwartz, Linebarger, Martin, & Bochetto, n.d.), and the Northwestern University (NWU) sentence comprehension test (Thompson, n.d.). The PCBA contrasts lexical (single-word) and sentence comprehension, semantically reversible and nonreversible sentence comprehension, and canonical and noncanonical sentence comprehension. This test also includes a grammaticality judgment subtest in which subjects listen to tape-recorded sentences, some of which contain grammatical errors, and determine whether they are "good" or "bad" sentences. The NWU sentences test examines comprehension of active,

passive, subject-relative, and object-relative sentences (20 exemplars of each). Semantically reversible picture pairs are presented and the patient points to the one that goes with target sentences.

Results of these tests showed that JD's lexical comprehension was superior to sentence comprehension and semantically reversible sentences were more difficult than nonreversible ones. JD also demonstrated better comprehension of active than passive sentences and grammaticality judgment was quite good. These findings were consistent with patterns of sentence comprehension seen in some agrammatic aphasic individuals (see Berndt et al., 1996).

3. **Sentence Production Testing.** Next, sentence production was analyzed in both constrained and narrative discourse conditions. This involved direct testing of verb and verb argument structure as well as production of several types of sentences. Narrative language samples also were collected, transcribed, and analyzed.

   a. **Verb and verb-argument structure production.** Testing production of verb and verb argument structure is important in assessing sentence production deficits. Without a verb, a word string cannot be considered a sentence. In addition, verbs are acquired together with knowledge about the participants that go into the "action" described by a verb. For example, when the verb *fix* is learned, it is learned that something must be fixed and that someone must do the fixing. This information, or the *arguments,* of the verb is typically represented in sentences by noun phrases (NPs) that occur in subject, object, and indirect object positions in sentences. Importantly, each argument of a verb is assigned a *thematic role* (e.g., Agent, Theme, Goal). The verb *fix* has two arguments, or thematic roles, therefore, it is a two-place verb. The verb *put* has three; therefore, it is a three-place verb (see Table 6–1).

   The argument structure properties of verbs are very important for sentence production, in that they must be observed in the syntax for sentences to be grammatical. For example, sentences such as **Zack fixed* or **Zack put the car* are ungrammatical because some of the arguments of the verbs are missing.

   JD was administered a verb production test battery with four subtests: verb comprehension, confrontation naming, elicited naming, and sentence production (Thompson, Lange, Schneider, & Shapiro, 1997). Several different types of verbs were

thief   artist   thief   artist

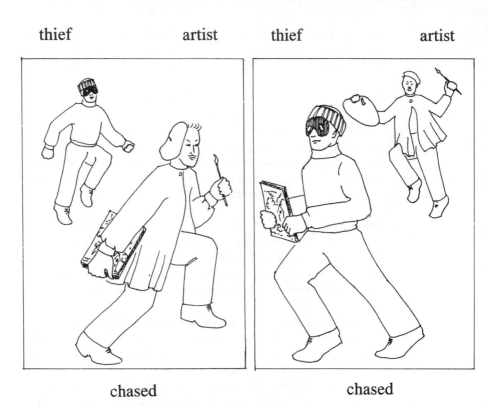

chased   chased

Figure 6–1. Sample picture stimuli used in sentence production priming task. The examiner presents a picture pair (one depicting the target sentence and the other a semantically reversed foil). Target sentence types (e.g., wh-questions, object clefts) are modeled using the foil picture and the subject is instructed to produce the target sentence type for the target picture.

tested for both comprehension and naming, including one-place verbs such as *sleep,* two-place verbs such as *fix,* three-place verbs such as *give,* and complement verbs such as *know,* which can be produced with either an NP or with a complement clause following the verb. Action pictures depicting each verb were used. To assess comprehension, JD was asked to point to the verb named (out of four pictures), and to assess confrontation naming, he was asked to name the action in individual pictures. Elicited naming involved the use of story completion cues. This subtest was included primarily for testing complement verbs which are difficult to picture. To elicit verbs in sentences arrows were added to the pictures to denote objects or people that represented arguments of the verb, and story completion cues were used to further constrain production.

Results showed that JD's verb comprehension was unimpaired. However, only 57% and 66% of verbs were produced correctly on confrontation naming and elicited naming subtests, respectively; and only 48% of sentences were produced correctly. Sentences with one- or two-place verbs were produced correctly more often than those with three-place or complement verbs. JD produced 85% of Agents, 65% of Patients/Themes, only 20% of Goals/Locations, and no complement clauses correctly.

b. **Simple and complex sentence production.** Production of active, passive, subject-relative clause, and object-relative clause sentences was tested using a sentence-production priming task (see Thompson, Shapiro et al., 1997). This task entailed presentation of a pair of pictures, one depicting the target sentence and the other depicting its semantically reversed counterpart (see Figure 6–1). The examiner elicited sentences by modeling the target sentence type using the semantically reversed picture and then asking JD to produce a similar sentence using the target picture. JD had most difficulty with production of passive sentences (20% correct) and object relatives (0% correct), with better production of subject relatives (50% correct) and actives (78% correct). He mis-ordered words and often produced the active form in attempts to produce complex sentences.

4. Discourse Analysis

a. **Collecting the language sample.** Narrative discourse samples were collected by asking JD to tell the stories of *Cinderella* and *Little Red Riding Hood*. Samples were transcribed and segmented into utterances based on syntactic, prosodic, and semantic criteria.

b. **Analyzing the sample.**
(1) **linguistic aspects.** Lexical and morphosyntactic patterns of narrative productions were analyzed using a method developed by Thompson, Shapiro, Tait et al. (1995). Results revealed an MLU of 2.23. Most utterances (i.e., 99%) were simple S-V-O sentences and of these only 8% were grammatically correct. Lexical analysis showed an open- to

closed-class word ratio of 3.0, indicating that for every three open-class words he produced one closed-class word.[3] He also produced more nouns than verbs with a noun to verb ratio of 1.78[4]. Errors in the closed class consisted primarily of deletion or substitution of auxiliary verbs, verb tense markers, and prepositions.

When verb productions were analyzed by type, we found a pattern similar to that derived from verb testing in the constrained production task. Eighty-six percent of the verbs produced were one- and two-place verbs; JD produced no three-place verbs, 8% were complement verbs, and 4% were copulas. Argument structure production in discourse also was impaired. Only 31% of his verbs were produced with correct argument structure.

(2) **communicative informativeness and efficiency.** Another important aspect of discourse analysis is to examine how well information is communicated to listeners—in spite of grammatical deficits. Therefore, JD's discourse samples were evaluated for communicative informativeness (i.e., the amount of information conveyed) and communicative efficiency (i.e., the rate at which information was conveyed). The method advanced by Nicholas and Brookshire (1993) was modified for use with *Cinderella* and *Red Riding Hood* stories using guidelines described by Jacobs (1996). The procedure involved a simple counting of correct information units (CIUs). The proportion of correct CIUs in the sample was computed by dividing the number of correct information units by the number of words. The number of CIUs produced per minute was calculated by dividing total CIUs by time.

In a sample of 200 words, 68 correct information units were produced in 6.5 minutes of narrative discourse. Thus, JD's speech production rate was 30.8 words per minute with only 10.5 CIUs produced per minute.

5. **Testing Functional Communication.** Finally, functional communication was tested using the American Speech-Language-Hearing Association *Functional Assessment of Communication Skills for*

---

[3]Normal subjects show open-class to closed-class ratio of .91 ($SD = 0.08$) in the same narrative conditions (Thompson et al., 1995).

[4]Normal subjects show noun to verb ratios of 1.21 ($SD = 0.25$) in the same narrative conditions (Thompson et al., 1995).

Adults (ASHA FACS; Frattali, Thompson, Holland, Wohl, & Fer-ketic, 1995), which tests the effects of communication impairments on everyday activities. The test includes both quantitative ratings reflecting communication independence, and qualitative ratings reflecting the quality of responses (the former a 7-point scale, the latter a 5-point scale). Quantitative performance is anchored at its low end by "does not do" and at its upper end by "does," with points between reflecting the relative amount of assistance needed to perform the communicative activity. Forty-three activities from four communication domains are assessed including (a) social communication, (b) communication of basic needs, (c) reading, writing, and number concepts, and (d) daily planning. Qualitative ratings reflect adequacy, appropriateness, promptness, and communication sharing.

Results showed an overall communication independence mean score of 5.8, with a range across domains of 4.7 (social communication) to 7.0 (daily planning). His overall qualitative dimension mean score was 3.61; promptness of responding and communication sharing were the most compromised with scores of 2.25 and 2.5, respectively. Most of JD's responses were adequate and appropriate.

IV. DIAGNOSIS

A. The Disorder: Summary of JD's Test Performance

Review of JD's test data indicated a performance pattern consistent with a diagnosis of Broca's aphasia with agrammatism. WAB and PICA scores indicated a moderately severe deficit that primarily affected verbal production, although deficits in other language modalities also were apparent. Comprehension testing indicated good ability to comprehend single words, including verbs, and conjoined commands; however, he had difficulty comprehending noncanonical, semantically reversed sentences.

Verbal production was limited to simple sentences, most of which were grammatically ill-formed. Main verbs were often missing and when he did produce verbs, he often failed to produce the verb's correct arguments, produced arguments in the wrong order, and/or deleted auxiliary verbs and tense markers. His production fit the pattern of Tissot et al.'s (1973) grammatical impairment Type 3: He rarely produced complete, grammatical sentences, but production of most (but not all) grammatical morphemes was spared.

His grammatical impairment also affected some aspects of functional communication, in particular social communication. The number of information units produced was quite low, his responses often were delayed, and he relied heavily on his communication partners in conversation. However, in spite of his deficits, he performed well in activities that required simple verbal responses or nonverbal responses.

B. Considerations for Treatment

It was determined that JD might benefit from treatment focused on sentence production. Although he might also have benefited from sentence comprehension treatment, his production difficulty affected his communication more than his comprehension deficit, and he desired to improve his sentence production abilities.

Because of the central role that verbs play in sentence production, and because JD presented with sentence production deficits characterized by problems with verb and verb argument structure production, we began with treatment focused on production of verbs in simple, active sentences. We emphasized the argument structure properties of verbs and the thematic roles of noun phrases that express argument structure. We also planned to extend treatment to complex sentence production, again emphasizing verb argument structure and the way that arguments are moved out of their canonical position when complex sentences are formed. We surmised that this treatment would further enhance production of grammatical sentences.

V. PROGNOSIS

A. Prognostic Signs

Prognosis for improvement was favorable. Although JD was 2 years postonset of stroke, he had shown marked improvement since onset and the improvement had been steady. Also, we have successfully treated sentence production deficits in other individuals who were several years postonset. In addition, JD was young, well educated, and very motivated to improve.

B. Expected Outcome

It was predicted that treatment would improve production of verbs and verb argument structure, and that this improvement would translate to greater usage of grammatical sentences in discourse. We also expected a shift from simple to more complex sentence production, although complex sentence production treatment was prescribed to enhance access to verbs and verb arguments structure, not to increase production of complex sentences per se. We also predicted that training production of complex sentences might improve comprehension of complex sentences. Finally, we expected treatment to influence functional communication by increasing the content, informativeness, and speed of communication.

VI. FOCUSING THE TREATMENT

A. Methods

1. **Treatment I. Verb and Verb Argument Structure Treatment.** Verb and verb argument structure treatment involved training production of two- and three-place verbs in sentences (see Appendix 6–A for details). NP-V-NP-PP sentences were developed for each of the verbs. The prepositional phrases (PPs) used with the two-place verbs were adjuncts; whereas those used with three-place verbs were arguments. The three-place verbs included both alternating and nonalternating datives; alternating datives were also targeted in NP-V-NP-NP form.

   Action picture stimuli were developed for each of 50 target sentences and used to elicit their production. Production of all sentences was tested prior to treatment in five separate baseline sessions over 2 weeks.

   JD was first trained to produce sentences with two-place verbs and adjunct prepositional phrases. Following this, he was trained to produce three-place alternating verbs in NP-V-NP-NP sentences. The action pictures, a set of cards on which the sentence constituents for target sentences were written, and an icon board were used in treatment (see Figure 6–2). Sentence constituents (e.g., the action, Agent-of-the-action) were individually identified and JD was required to place them in their corresponding slots on the icon board. He then practiced producing derived sentences.

   JD was seen for two, 1-hour sessions per week. Each training sentence was practiced at least twice. Production of all sentences was tested weekly to examine learning and generalization patterns. JD received a total of 10 weeks of this treatment (5 weeks for each of two sentence types).

2. **Treatment II. Training Complex Sentence Production.** The second treatment involved production of complex, noncanonical sen-

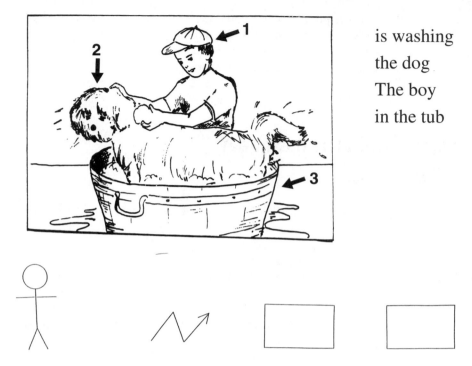

is washing
the dog
The boy
in the tub

Figure 6–2. Sample icon board used for verb and verb argument structure treatment. Picture taken from the PCBA (Saffran et al., n.d.)

tences in which sentence constituents have been moved out of their subject-verb-object order. Formation of noncanonical sentences requires movement of sentence constituents from d-structure (an underlying form) to s-structure[5]. This transformation is referred to by Chomsky (1991, 1993) as *move-alpha*. Consider the following:

1. Who$_i$ did Zack kiss$_{trace\ i}$?

The wh-question in (1) is formed by moving *who* from its original site, the direct object position, to the sentence initial position. This movement leaves a *trace* behind in the original position of *who*. Importantly, the thematic roles of the verb are assigned before movement occurs and, thus, when *who* is moved, it retains its thematic role—in this case the role of *Patient*.

---

[5]The terms *deep structure* and *surface structure* have been replaced by d- and s-structure, respectively, in Chomsky's more recent writings.

Similar movement operations are involved in sentences such as:

2. It was Bria$_i$ who Zack kissed$_{trace\ i}$. (object cleft)
3. Bria$_i$ was kissed$_{trace\ i}$ by Zack. (passive)

In (2) and (3) the direct object NP is moved from its original post verbal position—where its thematic role is received—and a trace of its movement is left behind. Thus, despite appearing in different grammatical positions, the thematic roles of sentence NPs in (1), (2), and (3) are the same: *Zack* is the Agent and *Bria* (or *who* in (1)) is the Patient.

There are two major types of phrasal movement: *wh*-movement and NP-movement. *Wh*-movement is involved in wh-questions, relative clauses, and object clefts; NP-movement occurs in the derivation of passives and NP-raising structures (e.g., *Zack seems to have kissed Bria*).

a. **Training *wh*-movement structures: Wh-questions.** In this phase of treatment, JD was trained to produce *wh*-questions (see Appendix 6–B). As discussed above, formation of *wh*-questions involves moving sentence elements from d-structure to s-structure via *wh*-movement. Four wh-question types were selected for training: *who, what, when,* and *where* and 20 target questions were developed for each. Importantly, *who*- and *what*-questions are formed by movement of the object NP (argument movement); and *where*- and *when*-questions are formed by moving an adjunct phrase (adjunct movement).

The active declarative counterpart of each question was used for both testing and treatment of wh-question production. These NP-V-NP-PP sentences contained the same lexical information (and, crucially, the same thematic role assignments) as the target wh-questions. For example, for the question, *Who is the soldier pushing into the street?*, the following declarative sentence was prepared.

4. The soldier is pushing the woman into the street.

Prior to treatment, JD's ability to produce all question types was tested twice in a 1-week baseline period. The active declarative sentences were presented in written form and instructions for producing each question type were provided.

JD then was trained to produce target wh-questions using a series of steps that emphasized the lexical and syntactic properties of the declarative sentence form as well as the *wh*-movement required to derive the surface realization of target wh-questions. A set of training cards on which individual sentence constituents were written (i.e., NPs, auxiliary verbs, verbs with -ing inflection, and PPs) were used for treatment. Additional cards containing the single words *who, what, where,* and *when* were also used. One wh-question type was trained at a time (i.e., *when*-questions were trained first) until all had been trained or until generalized production to untrained question types occurred. Treatment for each wh-question type was provided for 10 training sessions. Prior to every other treatment session, production of all 80 wh-questions was tested using procedures identical to baseline.

b. **Training *wh*- and NP-movement structures.** In the final phase of treatment, JD was trained to produce both *wh*- and NP-movement structures (see Appendix 6–B). *Wh*-movement structures included who-questions and object clefts and NP-movement sentences included passives and subject raising structures. These sentences were trained using a set of 15 active sentences of the form NP-V-NP. All sentences were semantically reversible with animate nouns. Each sentence was paired with a picture stimulus. A picture stimulus also was developed to represent the semantically reversible counterpart of each sentence. See Figure 6–1.

During baseline, verbal production of the four sentence types was tested using the sentence production priming task described previously. During each baseline probe session, the 15 picture pairs were presented in random order four times each (once to elicit each of the four sentence types), for a total of 60 sentence productions per probe.

Training procedures were similar to those for wh-questions. First, a picture pair was presented and JD was given the opportunity to produce the target sentence using the sentence production priming task. Next, the target picture was presented together with sentence constituent stimulus cards representing the active form of the target sentence, such as:

5. [The thief] [chased] [the artist]

Grammatical elements required in the s-structure of target sentences types (e.g., *it was, who, by, has, to have*) also were displayed. The examiner then identified the verb, the subject, and object NPs and explained their roles in relation to the verb. The movement operations required to formulate target sentences then were demonstrated.

JD received treatment of this type two times per week. Prior to every other training session, the complete set of 60 sentences was tested as in baseline. During training sessions, each sentence was practiced at least once, and not more than three times. JD received a total of 20 sessions for each sentence type.

B. Outcome Measures

Several outcome measures were used. As described above, baseline and treatment probes were administered prior to and throughout treatment of all sentence types. In addition, several measures administered during the initial examination were re-administered following Treatment I and once again following Treatment II. These included the WAB, the PCBA, the verb production battery, and the ASHA FACS (the PICA was administered following Treatment I only). Narrative samples also were collected and analyzed at each treatment interval.

VII. RESULTS

A. Progress on Targeted Behaviors

1. **Effects of Verb and Verb-Argument Structure Production Treatment.** JD's performance on verb and verb argument structure training is shown in Figure 6–3. As can be seen, he had great difficulty producing any of the verb types in sentences with their arguments/adjuncts prior to treatment. When sentences with two-place verbs and adjuncts were trained, JD quickly acquired the ability to produce them. Sentences with three-place alternating verbs in the form of NP-V-NP-NP were then targeted and JD's production of this sentence type improved.

    a. **Generalization and maintenance.** Also shown in Figure 6–3 are generalization data. When JD was trained to produce sentences with two-place verbs and adjuncts, generalization to three-place verbs in the form of NP-V-NP-PP also was seen.

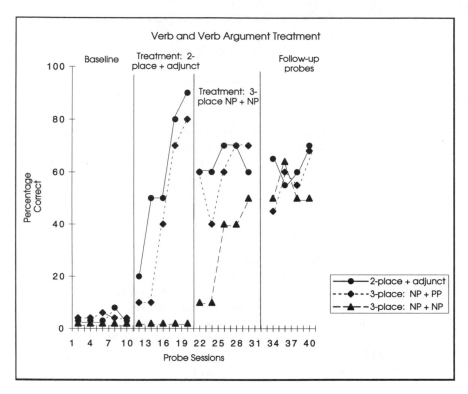

Figure 6–3. Percentage correct production of two-place and three-place verbs in sentence contexts during baseline and verb and verb argument structure treatment phases

However, no change in NP-V-NP-NP forms occurred. Follow-up probes administered at 2, 3, 4, and 5 weeks posttreatment indicated that JD retained the ability to produce all sentence forms at levels much higher than baseline.

2. **Effects of Training Complex *Wh*-Movement Sentences: Wh-questions.** JD's performance on sentence production probes during baseline and treatment of wh-questions is shown in Figure 6–4. Results indicated that treatment improved production of wh-questions. Production of all wh-questions was stable during baseline testing and improved when treatment was applied.

   a. **Generalization to untrained wh-questions.** An interesting pattern was seen in JD's generalization data—a pattern that we have noted in other patients who have received this treatment. When treatment was applied to *when*-questions, requiring

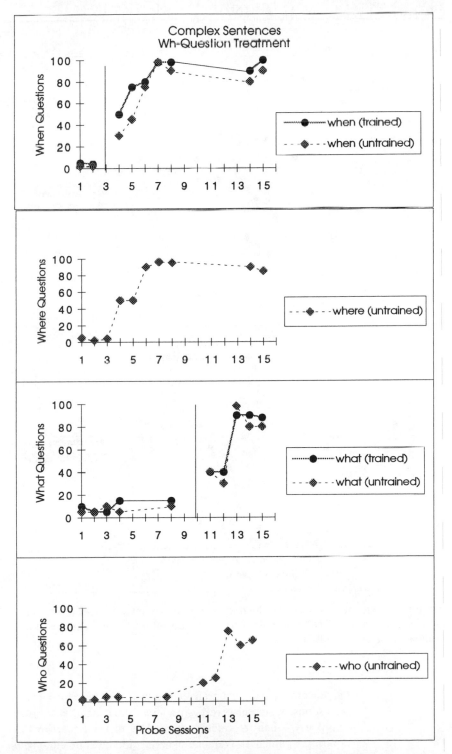

Figure 6–4. Percentage grammatically correct and complete wh-questions produced during baseline and wh-question treatment phases

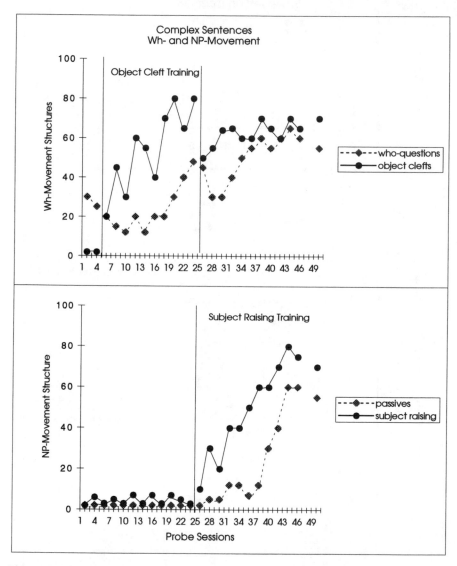

Figure 6–5. Percentage correct production of wh-movement structures (object clefts and who-questions) and NP-movement structures (subject-raising and passives) during baseline and treatment phases

adjunct movement, generalized production of untrained *where*-questions, which also rely on adjunct movement, was noted. Similarly, when treatment was applied to *what*-questions requiring argument movement, generalization was noted to *who-*

questions. Importantly, adjunct movement did not generalize to argument movement constructions. Examination of sentence production error patterns also was interesting. In early phases of treatment, JD evinced primary difficulty coreferencing the *wh* word with the moved sentence constituent, that is, he produced both the *wh*-word *and* its counterpart and seemed not to realize that they both conveyed the same thematic roles. For example, he produced responses such as: "*Who* is the soldier pushing *the woman*?" for the target: "Who$_i$ is the soldier pushing t$_i$ into the street?"; or "*Where* is the soldier pushing *into the street*?" for the target: "Where$_i$ is the soldier pushing the woman t^i?" Later probes indicated that this problem was eliminated.

b. **Maintenance.** Maintenance of wh-question production was tested at four and six weeks post treatment. These data indicated that JD retained the ability to produce targeted wh-questions on the probe task.

3. **Effects of Training Complex *Wh*- and NP-Movement Structures.** Data representing correct *wh*- and NP-movement structures during baseline and treatment probes for JD are shown in Figure 6–5. These data indicated that during the baseline phase production of all sentence types was poor, although who-questions were produced at a higher level than the other sentence types, as JD had previously received treatment on wh-question production. During baseline, JD once again produced errors of coreference. Also, he often produced active sentences or did not respond.

Following baseline testing, successful acquisition of treated sentence types was noted. During object cleft training, production of object clefts improved over baseline levels, ranging from 20% to 80% correct. Importantly, object cleft training did not influence production of passive or subject-raising structures. Subsequent training of subject-raising structures resulted in improved production of this sentence type with performance ranging from 10% to 80% correct production.

a. **Generalization across sentence types.** Training JD to produce object cleft sentences, which rely on *wh*-movement, influenced production of *who* questions that also rely on *wh*-movement. *Who* question production improved from 30% during baseline to a high of 48% during object cleft training;

however, training object clefts did not influence production of passives or subject-raising structures (see object cleft training phase in Figure 6–5). This pattern of performance was perhaps a result of his previous wh-question treatment or it may have been because object clefts and wh-questions are linguistically related.

Generalization from trained NP-movement structures (subject-raising structures) to untrained NP-movement structures (passives) also was noted. Untrained passive sentences improved from 0% correct to 60% correct during training of subject-raising structures (see subject-raising training phase in Figure 6–5).

b. **Maintenance.** A follow-up probe was administered 3 weeks after the completion of treatment. Production of both *wh-* and NP-movement structures was maintained.

B. Performance on Aphasia Test Batteries

Performance on the WAB and the PICA on pretesting, following completion of Treatment I, and following Treatment II, when complex sentence structures were trained, is shown in Table 6–2. Little change in WAB or PICA performance was seen from pretesting to post-Treatment I. This finding was not surprising, as the time from between testings was only 20 weeks. Improvements in performance, however, were noted on the final administration of the WAB, given approximately 1 year later. Notably, JD's aphasia quotient increased from 62 at pretreatment to 75 at post-Treatment II. JD's fluency score remained at 4, however, information content improved. Improvements also were noted on naming and comprehension subtests. Due to time constraints the PICA was not re-administered.

C. Performance on Sentence Comprehension

Sentence comprehension was tested at all test intervals using the PCBA. Results of this testing also are shown in Table 6–2. From pretesting to post-Treatment I, overall sentence comprehension improved from 78% correct to 82% correct. Improved scores also were noted on grammaticality judgment. On post-Treatment II testing, scores on sentence comprehension further improved, with overall performance increasing to 88% correct. Notably, reversible sentence comprehension improved from 63% to 88% correct, and improved scores were also derived for noncanonical, passive, and object-relative sentences.

Table 6-2. Performance on aphasia test batteries, tests of auditory comprehension, and tests of verb and verb argument structure production at pretreatment, posttreatment I, and following completion of Treatment II

Tests administered	Pretreatment	Posttreatment I	Posttreatment II
Western Aphasia Battery			
Aphasia quotient	62	64	75
Fluency	4/10	4/10	4/10
Information content	7/10	7/10	9/10
Comprehension	8/10	8/10	9.5/10
Repetition	5/10	6/10	6/10
Naming	7/10	7/10	9/10
Reading	7/10	8/10	8/10
Porch Index of			
Communicative Abilities			
Overall percentile	72	75	
Gestural percentile	71	75	
Verbal percentile	59	62	
Graphic percentile	77	76	
Philadelphia Comprehension			
Battery for Aphasia (percentage			
correct)			
Lexical comprehension	100	100	100
Grammaticality judgment	85	93	92
Sentence comprehension	78	82	88
Reversible	54	63	88
Lexical	95	100	100
Active	90	95	100
Subject relative	85	85	85
Passive/object relative	50	60	70
Verb Production Battery			
(Percentage Correct)			
Confrontation naming	57	87	92
One-place	65	95	
Two-place	60	89	
Three-place	41	57	
Compliment	65	86	
Elicited naming	66	85	98
One-place	75	92	
Two-place	68	70	
Three-place	55	64	
Compliment	65	86	
Sentence production	48	74	88
One-place	80	84	
Two-place	65	84	
Three-place	60	56	
Compliment	40	63	
Argument structure types			
Agents	85	94	100
Patient/theme	65	84	94
Goal/location	20	50	80
Complement clause	00	29	60

D. Changes on Sentence Production Measures

To examine changes in sentence production, verb and verb argument structure production was tested using our verb production battery and narrative discourse samples were collected and analyzed as in pretesting.

1. **Changes in Verb and Verb Argument Structure Production.** Results indicated marked improvement in production of verbs following Treatment I, with total correct verb production increasing from 57% to 87% correct on the verb and verb argument structure production test (see Table 6–2). Notably, this improvement was seen across all verb types. Verb production also continued to improve throughout complex sentence production treatment. On posttesting, JD produced 92% of verbs correctly in confrontation naming; 98% were produced correctly in the elicited production condition.

   Improved sentence production ability also was noted with increases from 48% correct to 74% correct following Treatment I and from 74% to 88% correct following Treatment II.

2. **Results of Narrative Language Sample Analysis**

   a. **Linguistic changes in the discourse.** Narrative language sample data collected at pretreatment, following verb and verb argument structure treatment and following complex sentence production treatment are presented in Table 6–3. These data revealed several changes over time in linguistic aspects of JD's narrative discourse. Mean length of utterance increased from 2.23 to 4.85 and the proportion of JD's sentences that were considered grammatical increased from 8% at pretesting to 39% on the final sample. Also, a shift from production of primarily simple sentences to production of complex ones was noted during complex sentence production treatment. Open-class to closed-class ratios also improved, although he continued to produce more open- than closed-class words on final testing. Noun to verb ratio also improved.

   The most notable changes in JD's discourse reflected improvement in verb and verb argument structure production. At pretreatment, only 31% of the verbs were produced with correct arguments around them. Whereas, following Treatment I, correct argument structures were produced for 52% of verbs. Continued improvement was seen during Treatment II; on final

Table 6-3. Production patterns found in JD's narrative discourse at pre-treatment, following Treatment I, and in post-Treatment II samples

	Pretreatment	Posttreatment I	Posttreatment II
Number of words	200	250	358
MLU	2.23	3.20	4.85
Linguistic Variables			
Grammatical sentences	.08	.18	.39
Simple sentences	.99	.74	.54
Complex sentences	.01	.26	.46
Noun/verb	1.78	1.03	1.09
Open-class/closed-class	3.00	3.00	2.32
Verbs produced by type			
One-place	.44	.18	.03
Two-place	.42	.25	.05
Three-place	.00	.03	.00
Complement	.08	.37	.66
Copula	.04	.07	.04
Correct argument structure production			
One-place	.40	.62	1.00
Two-place	.36	.52	.69
Three-place	.00	.00	.50
Complement	.40	.46	.40
Copula	.70	.85	1.00
Total verbs with correct arguments	.31	.52	.60
Informativeness and efficiency			
Number of CIUs	68	103	139
Time	6.50	6.10	6.90
Words per minute	30.80	40.90	51.90
Proportion of CIUs	.34	.41	.39
Information units per minute	10.50	16.80	20.10

Note: CIU = Correct Information Unit

testing, 60% of verbs were produced with correct argument structure.

b. **Changes in communicative informativeness and efficiency.** Table 6–3 also presents data on communicative informativeness and efficiency. As can be seen, improvement over time was noted, not only in the number of words produced per minute, but also in the proportion of CIUs produced per minute. These data indicated that improvements noted in lin-

Table 6–4. ASHA FACS data from pre- and post-treatment administrations

	Pretreatment	*Posttreatment*
Communication Domains		
Social communication	4.70	6.09
Communication of basic needs	5.00	6.70
Reading, writing, number concepts	6.80	6.90
Daily planning	7.00	7.00
Overall communication independence mean score	5.80	6.67
Qualitative Dimensions		
Adequacy	4.70	5.00
Appropriateness	5.00	5.00
Promptness	2.25	4.25
Communication sharing	2.50	3.00
Overall qualitative dimension mean score	3.61	4.30

guistic aspects of production translated to improvements in the amount of information conveyed and in the efficiency of communication.

E. The Effects of Treatment on Functional Communication

We administered the ASHA FACS both prior to and following the completion of treatment to examine the influence of sentence production treatment on JD's ability to communicate functionally. Results are shown in Table 6–4. As predicted, improvements in both quantitative and qualitative aspects of functional communication were noted across testing periods. As might have been expected, most improvement was noted in the areas of social communication; however, we also saw improvement in communication of basic needs and in functional writing ability.

VIII. DISCUSSION

A. Reasons for Treatment Effects Noted

There are two potential reasons for the noted improvement in JD's sentence production ability. One concerns the aspects of sentence production that were trained and the other concerns the manner in which they were trained. JD's sentence constructional deficits were characterized by difficulty in producing verbs and in selecting and ordering the arguments of the verb in sentences. This difficulty greatly influenced his ability to produce grammatical sentences and therefore these aspects of sentence production were selected for treatment. It was necessary to consider the lexical properties of verbs selected for treatment and to consider the syntactic properties of sentences in which the verbs were trained. Also, the generalization effects that were seen across sentences largely resulted from carefully selecting structures with similar lexical and syntactic properties for generalization analysis.

In addition, the linguistic properties of sentences were considered in the design of the treatment provided. JD showed good ability to comprehend both nouns and verbs, his active sentence comprehension was good, and he performed well on grammaticality judgment. We therefore surmised that he had at least some access to verbs and thematic information, but he did not use them fully in his sentence productions nor did he assign thematic roles normally in complex sentences. Therefore, it was important to begin treatment with tasks concerned with establishing and improving knowledge and access to the thematic role information around verbs. This was accomplished in Treatment I. Next, the operations involved in establishing co-reference among elements in complex sentences, that is, establishing that the thematic information of verbs is represented in all sentences, but that the sentence constituents representing that thematic information may appear in various places in sentences, was thought to be important. This part of the treatment was not provided to enhance production of trained sentence types so much as it was to further enhance knowledge about the lexical representation of verbs and how this translates to production of grammatical sentences of any type.

Probe task results showed that our goals were accomplished, and we saw evidence of treatment efficacy on both our verb production battery and also in narrative discourse. Clearly, on both tasks, JD showed improved access to verb production and, in turn, improved ability to produce argument structures in sentences. He also produced an increased proportion of grammatical sentences and showed improvements in sentence comprehension. We attribute these changes to the treatment, which we believe enhanced JD's access to the essential structural elements of grammatical sentences. It is important to point out, however, that the tests which we used to examine sentence production and comprehension are not standardized measures and, therefore, test-retest effects are unknown.

Improvement was also noted on functional outcome measures such as communicative informativeness and efficiency and, importantly, on the AHSA FACS. These changes were not surprising. Indeed, treatment that results in improved access to the grammar should also result in increases in communicative informativeness, efficiency, and ability to functionally communicate. If such effects had not been forthcoming, the treatment provided for JD might have been deemed ineffective.

B. Limitations and Some Alternative Approaches

Some comments are warranted in terms of the limitations of the treatment provided for JD. He remains agrammatic. In spite of JD's somewhat remarkable recovery of language, all of JD's language deficits were not remediated. He continues to evince difficulty with auxiliary verbs and with bound verb morphology, his utterances remain shorter and less complex than normal, and his speech remains effortful. JD needs further treatment to address these deficits. Some promising treatments aimed at improving access to verb morphology in both spoken and written language have recently been reported (see, for example, Mitchum, 1992; Mitchum, Haendiges, & Berndt, 1993). JD might benefit from these.

Would JD have benefited more if a different approach to treatment of the structural aspects of his sentence deficits had been applied? Even though treatment for sentence production deficits seen in agrammatic aphasia has received little attention in the literature, there are a few available alternatives. These fall into two categories: (a) those that apply treatment directly to the types of sentences that are observed to be problematic for the patient (e.g., wh-questions, passives) (Helm-Estabrooks & Albert, 1991; Thompson & McReynolds, 1986; Wambaugh & Thompson, 1989), and (b) those that attempt to enhance access to lexical and syntactic aspects of sentences (Byng, 1988; Jones, 1986; Loverso, Prescott, & Selinger, 1986; Schwartz, Saffran, Fink, Myers, & Martin, 1994; Thompson et al., 1993; Thompson, Shapiro, Ballard, Jacobs, Schneider, & Tait, 1997; Thompson, Shapiro, Tait, Jacobs, & Schneider, 1996). Research examining the effects of the former has shown that subjects improve in their ability to produce trained sentences. However, less impressive findings have been reported with regard to generalization. For example, we (Thompson & McReynolds, 1986) trained four agrammatic aphasic individuals to produce *what*-questions and, although all subjects improved, training did not influence production of *who-*, *where-*, or *when*-questions. In addition, this treatment had no effect on the subjects' narrative production. It is likely that JD would have performed similarly had he been provided with a direct production approach; that is, he probably would not have generalized across sentence types or to narrative discourse.

This noted lack of generalization when using direct production approaches led researchers to take a different—more theoretical—direction in developing treatment methods for sentence production deficits. Instead of focusing directly on the surface representation of sentences, these treatments focus on aspects of production (or processing) that are thought be awry in agrammatic aphasia. For example, Loverso and colleagues (Loverso et al., 1986) developed a method known as "verb as core" treatment, which is quite similar to the verb and verb argument structure treatment that JD was provided.

Another treatment for improving both comprehension and production of sentences is mapping therapy (Byng, 1988; Jones, 1986; Schwartz et al., 1994). Mapping therapy, developed to help agrammatic patients overcome problems with mapping thematic (semantic) information onto the syntax, also focuses on training patients to recognize the thematic roles of sentence NPs in simple, active, canonical sentences and in more complex, noncanonical sentences. Subjects treated using this method have improved their comprehension of both canonical and noncanonical sentence forms and have demonstrated changes in narrative production patterns. However, as with direct production approaches, improvement has been limited largely to sentence types used in treatment. It is likely that JD would have benefited from both "verb as core" and mapping therapy approaches. It is unknown, however, which of these might have been most efficacious. Controlled studies are needed comparing the effects of various treatments for agrammatism.

It also is possible that JD would have benefited more from training complex aspects of the grammar prior to training simpler ones. For example, training complex sentences first might have resulted in generalization to verb and verb argument structure production in active sentences, and therefore eliminated the need for direct verb and verb argument structure treatment. Although training complex language prior to training simple language structures is counterintuitive, recent data from my lab have indicated positive generalization to structures that are in a subset relation to the structures trained. For example, training agrammatic subjects to produce object clefts (which contain an embedded clause) results in generalization to who-questions that do not. However, generalization to object clefts does not appear to result from training who-questions. Similar effects have been noted in studies using computer-simulated language networks. When established networks are damaged, retraining more complex (or less representative) exemplars from a category results in greater generalization than retraining less complex (i.e., more prototypical) exemplars (Plaut, 1996). Further research comparing the generalization effects of training simple versus complex aspects of language is needed in order to validate these observations.

C. Summary and Conclusion

In summary, the treatment provided for JD was effective. Not only did he show improvement in production of treated structures, he also improved in his production of untrained, linguistically related structures. In addition, treatment affected his aphasia in general as tested by the WAB, and he improved in both the linguistic structure and the content of his discourse. Finally, JD's data showed that treatment influenced aspects of functional communication.

It is important to point out that these changes were accomplished when JD was 2 years postonset, and that the improvements resulted from 1½ years of treatment. These findings indicate that important changes in language functioning can be accomplished several years poststroke, when the proper treatments are applied and when treatment is extended over a long period of time. Unfortunately, due to current health care policies in the United States, most patients like JD receive treatment for only a few sessions and sometimes for only a few weeks poststroke.

Further research is needed to examine (a) the effects of treatment such as that provided for JD in patients who are in early versus chronic stages of recovery, (b) the effects or various treatment approaches, and (c) the effects of shorter periods of treatment. It is possible, for example, that JD's sentence production would have improved more quickly if he had been provided with sentence production treatment very soon after the onset of his stroke, instead of the more traditional treatment that he received. However, it also is possible that the treatment provided in the early recovery period was needed to support recovery of sentence production. It also is possible that another type of treatment might have been more beneficial for JD or that shorter periods of treatment might have resulted in similar outcomes. It is suggested, however, that until such issues are clarified, patients showing agrammatic patterns like JD's be provided with treatment similar to that described here—even at early times poststroke and even if only a few treatment sessions are possible. The number of sessions devoted to each sentence type may be decreased, or sentence types may be trained in combination to cut down the number of treatment sessions. Home practice exercises also could be developed to coincide with in-clinic treatment, and family members or other volunteers could be recruited to assist. Future research will help to clarify the type and amount of treatment that will result in the greatest effects, and when in the course of recovery is the best time to provide it.

IX. ACKNOWLEDGMENTS

The work reported here was supported in part by the National Institutes on Deafness and Other Communication Disorders (NIDCD) grant DC01948.

X. REFERENCES

Berndt, R. S. (1987). Symptom co-occurrence and dissociation in the interpretation of agrammatism. In M. Coltheart, G. Sartori, & R. Job (Eds.), *The neuropsychology of language* (pp. 221–233). London: Erlbaum.

Berndt, R. S., Mitchum, C. C., & Haendiges, A. N. (1996). Comprehension of reversible sentences in "agrammatism": A meta-analysis. *Cognition, 58,* 289–308.

Bock, J. K. (1987). Co-coordinating words and syntax in speech plans. In A. W. Ellis (Ed.), *Progress in the psychology of language* (Vol. 3). London: Erlbaum.

Byng, S. (1988). Sentence processing deficits: Theory and therapy. *Cognitive Neuropsychology, 5,* 629–676.

Caplan, D., Baker, C., & Dehaut, F. (1985). Syntactic determinants of sentence comprehension in aphasia. *Cognition, 21,* 117–175.

Caplan, D., & Hanna, J. E. (in press). Sentence production by aphasic patients in a constrained task. *Brain and Language.*

Caramazza, A., & Hillis, A. E. (1989). The disruption of sentence production: Some dissociations. *Brain and Language, 35,* 625–650.

Chomsky, N. (1991). Some notes on economy of derivation and representation. In R. Freidin (Ed.), *Principles and parameters in comparative grammar* (pp. 415–454). Cambridge, MA: MIT Press.

Chomsky, N. (1993). A minimalist program for linguistic theory. In K. Hale & S. J. Keyser (Eds.), *The view from Building 20: Essays in linguistics in honor of Sylvain Bromberger* (pp. 1–51) Cambridge, MA: MIT Press.

deBlesser, R. (1987). From agrammatism to paragrammatism: German aphasiological traditions and grammatical disturbances. *Cognitive Neuropsychology, 4,* 187–256.

Fratalli, C., Thompson, C. K., Holland, A. L., Wohl, C. B., & Ferketic, M. (1995). *American Speech-Language-Hearing Association Functional Assessment of Communication Skills for Adults.* Rockville, MD: ASHA.

Garrett, M. F. (1980). Levels of processing in sentence production. In B. Butterworth (Ed.), *Language production* (Vol. 1) (pp. 177–220). London: Academic Press.

Garrett, M. F. (1984). The organization of processing structure for language production: Applications to aphasic speech. In D. Caplan, A. R. Lecours, & A. Smith (Eds.), *Biological perspectives on language* (pp. 172–193). Cambridge, MA: MIT Press.

Goodglass, H. (1976). Agrammatism. In H. Whitaker & H. A. Whitaker (Eds.), *Studies in neurolinguistics* (Vol. 1) (pp. 237–260). New York: Academic Press.

Goodglass, H., Christiansen, J. A., & Gallagher, R. (1993). Comparison of morphology and syntax in free narrative and structured tests: Fluent vs. nonfluent aphasics. *Cortex, 29,* 377–407.

Grodzinsky, Y. (1986). Language deficits and syntactic theory. *Brain and Language, 27,* 135–159.

Grodzinsky, Y. (1995). A restrictive theory of agrammatic comprehension. *Brain and Language, 50,* 27–51.

Heeschen, C. (1985). Agrammatism versus paragrammatism: A fictitious opposition. In M. L. Kean (Ed.), *Agrammatism* (pp. 207–248). New York: Academic Press.

Helm-Estabrooks, N. A., & Albert, M. L. (1991). *Manual of aphasia therapy.* San Antonio, TX: PRO-ED, Inc.

Jacobs, B. J. (1996, November). *Analysis of language structure and function in aphasic discourse.* Paper presented at the American Speech-Language-Hearing Association Annual Convention. Seattle, WA.

Jones, E. V. (1986). Building the foundations for sentence production in a nonfluent aphasic. *British Journal of Disorders of Communication, 21,* 63–82.

Kertesz, A. (1982). *The Western Aphasia Battery.* San Antonio, TX: The Psychological Corporation.

Kohn, S. E., Lorch, M. P., & Pearson, D. M. (1989). Verb finding in aphasia. *Cortex, 25,* 57–69.

Kolk, H. H. J., Van Grusven, J. J. F., & Keyser, A. (1985). On parallelism between production and comprehension in agrammatism. In M. L. Kean (Ed.), *Agrammatism* (pp. 165–206). Orlando, FL: Academic Press.

Linebarger, M. C., Schwartz, M. F., & Saffran, E. M. (1983). Sensitivity to grammatical structure in so-called agrammatic aphasics. *Cognition, 13,* 361–392.

Loverso, F., Prescott, T., & Selinger, M. (1986). Cueing verbs: A treatment strategy for aphasic adults. *Journal of Rehabilitation Research, 25,* 47–60.

Mauner, G., Fromkin, V., & Cornell, T. (1993). Comprehension and acceptability judgments in agrammatism: Disruption in the syntax of referential dependency. *Brain and Language, 45,* 340–370.

Menn, L. (1990). Agrammatism in English: Two case studies. In L. Menn & L. K. Obler (Eds.), *Agrammatic aphasia: Cross-language narrative sourcebook* (pp. 117–178). Baltimore, MD: John Benjamins.

Miceli, G., & Mazzuchi, A. (1990). The nature of speech production deficits in so-called agrammatic aphasia: Evidence from two Italian patients. In L. Menn & L. K. Obler (Eds.), *Agrammatic aphasia: Cross-language narrative sourcebook* (pp. 717–816). Baltimore, MD: John Benjamins.

Miceli, G., Silveri, M. C., Nocentini, U., & Caramazza, A. (1988). Patterns of dissociation in comprehension and production of nouns and verbs. *Aphasiology, 2,* 351–358.

Micelli, G., Silveri, M. C., Romani, C., & Caramazza, A. (1989). Variation in the pattern of omissions and substitutions of grammatical morphemes in the spontaneous speech of so-called agrammatic patients. *Brain and Language, 36,* 447–492.

Miceli, G., Silveri, M. C., Villa, C., & Caramazza, A. (1984). On the basis for the agrammatics' difficulty in producing main verbs. *Cortex, 20,* 207–220.

Mitchum, C. C. (1992). Treatment generalization and the application of cognitive neuropsychological models in aphasia therapy. In *Aphasia treatment: Current approaches and research opportunities* (NIDCD Monograph). Bethesda, MD: National Institutes of Health, NIDCD.

Mitchum, C. C., Haendiges, A. N., & Berndt, R. S. (1993). Model-guided treatment to improve written sentence production: A case study. *Aphasiology, 7,* 71–109.

Nespoulous, J. L., Dordain, M., Perron, C., Ska, B., Bub, D., Caplan, D., Mehler, J., & Lecours, A. R. (1988). Agrammatism in sentence production without comprehension deficits: Reduced availability of syntactic structures and/or grammatical morphemes: A case study. *Brain and Language, 33,* 273–295.

Nicholas, L. E., & Brookshire, R. H. (1993). A system for quantifying the informativeness and efficiency of the connected speech of adults with aphasia. *Journal of Speech and Hearing Research, 36,* 338–350.

Plaut, D. C. (1996). Relearning after damage in connectionist networks: Toward a theory of rehabilitation. *Brain and Language, 52,* 25–82.

Porch, B. E. (1973). *The Porch Index of Communicative Abilities: Administration, scoring, and interpretation.* Palo Alto, CA: Consulting Psychologists Press.

Saffran, E. M., Berndt, R. S., & Schwartz, M. F. (1989). The quantitative analysis of agrammatic production: Procedure and data. *Brain and Language, 37,* 440–479.

Saffran, E. M., Schwartz, M. F., Linebarger, M., Martin, N., & Bochetto, P. (n.d.). *The Philadelphia Comprehension Battery for Aphasia.*

Saffran, E. M., Schwartz, M. F., & Marin, O. S. M. (1980). The word order problem in agrammatism: Production. *Brain and Language, 10,* 263–280.

Schwartz, M. F., Linebarger, M. C., Saffran, E. M., & Pate, D. S. (1987). Syntactic transparency and sentence interpretation in aphasia. *Language and Cognitive Processes, 2,* 85–113.

Schwartz, M. F., Saffran, E. M., Fink, R. B., Myers, J. L., & Martin, N. (1994). Mapping therapy: A treatment programme for agrammatism. *Aphasiology, 8,* 19–54.

Thompson, C. K. (n.d.). *Northwestern University Sentence Comprehension Test.*

Thompson, C. K. (1996). Linguistic-specific sentence production treatment for agrammatic aphasia. *Topics in Stroke Rehabilitation, 3,* 60–85.

Thompson, C. K., Lange, K., Schneider, S., & Shapiro, L. P. (1997). Agrammatic and non-brain-damaged subjects' verb and verb argument production in constrained elicitation conditions. *Aphasiology, 11,* 473–490.

Thompson, C. K., & McReynolds, L. V. (1986). Wh-interrogative production in agrammatic aphasia: An experimental analysis of auditory-visual stimulation and direct-production treatment. *Journal of Speech and Hearing Research, 29,* 193–206.

Thompson, C. K., Shapiro, L. P., Ballard, K. J., Jacobs, B. J., Schneider, S. L., & Tait, M. E. (1997). Training and generalized production of *wh-* and NP-movement structures in agrammatic aphasia. *Journal of Speech and Hearing Research, 40,* 228–244.

Thompson, C. K., Shapiro, L., Li, L., & Schendel, L. (1995). Analysis of verbs and verb-argument structure: A method for quantification of aphasic language production. In P. Lemme (Ed.), *Clinical aphasiology* (Vol. 23) (pp. 121–140). Austin, TX: PRO-ED.

Thompson, C. K., Shapiro, L. P., & Roberts, M. (1993). Treatment of sentence production deficits in aphasia: A linguistic-specific approach to wh-interrogative training and generalization. *Aphasiology, 7,* 111–133.

Thompson, C. K., Shapiro, L. P., Tait, M. E., Jacobs, B. J., & Schneider, S. L. (1996). Training *wh*-question production in agrammatic aphasia: Analysis of argument and adjunct movement. *Brain and Language, 52,* 175–228.

Thompson, C. K., Shapiro, L. P., Tait, M., Jacobs, B., Schneider, S., & Ballard, K. (1995). A system for systematic analysis of agrammatic language production (abstract). *Brain and Language, 51,* 124–129.

Tissot, R. J., Maunin, G., & Lhermitte, F. (1973). *L'agrammatisme.* Brussels: Dessart.

Wambaugh, J. L., & Thompson, C. K. (1989). Training and generalization of agrammatic aphasic adults' *wh*-interrogative productions. *Journal of Speech and Hearing Disorders, 54,* 509–525.

Zingeser, L., & Berndt, R. S., (1990). Retrieval of nouns and verbs in agrammatism and anomia. *Brain and Language, 39,* 14–32.

A P P E N D I X

6-A

I. TREATMENT I: VERB AND VERB ARGUMENT STRUCTURE TREATMENT

A. Stimuli

Two-place verbs with adjunct PP (NP-V-NP-PP) ($N = 20$); e.g., The man is mowing the lawn in the summer.

Three-place, nonalternating verbs (NP-V-NP-PP) ($N = 10$); e.g., The woman is putting the trash in the bin.

Three-place, alternating verbs (NP-V-NP-PP) ($N = 10$); e.g., The man is giving the money to the teller.

Three-place, alternating verbs (NP-V-NP-NP) ($N = 10$); e.g., The man is giving the teller the money.

B. Baseline and Treatment Probe Procedure

All target sentences were randomized and tested using picture stimuli developed for each. Arrows were placed on the pictures to denote people and/or objects representing arguments of the verb and adjuncts. The following instructions were presented: "I will show you some pictures and a word that describes the action picture. Each picture has 3 arrows. The arrows indicate people, objects, places, and times that the action is occurring. These arrows are numbered. I want you to make a sentence using the action word and all of the people/things indicated by the arrows. You must use the people/things marked with arrows in the order that they are numbered." Feedback regarding the accuracy of responding was not provided, but encouragement was given.

C. Treatment Procedures

The major sentence constituents (e.g., Agent, action, Theme) of sentences designated for treatment were printed on cards. On each training trial, the sentence constituent cards, corresponding action pictures (with arrows and numbers), and an icon board were presented. The icon board was divided into four sections. Each section contained a sentence constituent slot—from left to right, one for the Agent, one for the action, one for the Patient/Theme, and one for the PP. Above each slot was a symbol indicating which sentence constituent belonged in the slot. (See Figure 6–2.)

The clinician explained: "These symbols represent the parts of the sentence you will make." The examiner then pointed to each icon on the icon board and identified it. The action icon was identified first. For example, for the sentence, *The boy is washing the dog in the tub,* the clinician said: "This symbol represents the action." The verb card then was selected and placed in the action slot as the examiner explained: "The action in this picture is *wash,* someone is washing something at some place/time." The remaining symbols and their corresponding sentence constituents then were reviewed in the order of subject, direct object, and adjunct prepositional phrase. The examiner explained: "This symbol represents a person" (pointing to the symbol and to the boy in the picture). "The boy is the person doing the washing" (the sentence constituent card was placed in the slot). "This symbol represents a thing" (pointing to the symbol and the thing in the picture). "The dog is the thing being washed" (the direct object sentence constituent card was placed in the corresponding slot). "And this symbol represents a place" (examiner points to symbol and the tub in the picture). "The tub is the place where the dog is being washed" (examiner placed the adjunct PP card in the appropriate slot). JD then was instructed to read the sentence aloud. The sentence constituent cards were removed from the slots, placed in random order on the side of the icon board, and JD was instructed to place the sentence constituent cards in their proper slots, one at a time, as the examiner again identified the thematic roles for each. When the cards were in correct order, JD was instructed to read the sentence aloud. Feedback and assistance were provided. A similar procedure was used for training NP-V-NP-NP structures.

A P P E N D I X

6-B

II. TREATMENT II: TRAINING COMPLEX SENTENCE PRODUCTION

A. *Wh*-Movement Structures (Wh-Questions)

1. Stimuli

Who and *what* questions (argument movement)
1. Who$_i$ is the soldier pushing t_i into the street? ($N = 20$)
2. What$_i$ is the boy kicking t_i in the barn? ($N = 20$)
   When and *where* questions (adjunct movement)
3. When$_i$ is the student helping the doctor t_i? ($N = 20$)
4. Where$_i$ is the guard protecting the clerk t_i? ($N = 20$)

2. Baseline and Treatment Probe Procedure.
The active, declarative form of target wh-questions were individually presented and JD was instructed to formulate a question for each. Specific instructions for eliciting each question type were given. Using, for example, the active sentence, *The soldier is pushing the woman into the street,* a *who*-question was elicited with the following instruction: "You want to know the person the soldier is pushing, so you ask?" The word *person* was emphasized and rising inflection was used. To elicit *what*-questions using a stimulus sentence such as *The boy is kicking the cow in the barn,* the examiner instructed: "You want

149

to know the thing the boy is kicking, so you ask?" This time, the word *thing* was emphasized. To elicit *when-* and *where-*questions, the same procedure was used except that JD was instructed to ask about the time or the place, respectively. JD was given approximately 10 seconds to produce each question response. If a response did not occur within the allotted 10-second period, a new stimulus was presented and instructions to ask another wh-question were provided. Feedback as to the accuracy of response was not given during this probe task, but intermittent encouragement was provided.

3. **Treatment Procedures.** Active, declarative sentences corresponding with target wh-questions were used in treatment in conjunction with a set of training cards on which individual sentence constituents were written (i.e., NPs, auxiliary verbs, verbs with -ing inflection, and PPs). Additional cards containing the single words *who, what, where,* and *when,* and a question mark card were also used. Treatment entailed a series of steps emphasizing the lexical and syntactic properties of the declarative sentence form as well as the *wh*-movement required to derive the surface realization of target wh-questions. For each active sentence, JD was trained to (a) recognize the verb, verb argument structure, and thematic roles of NPs, (b) move the proper sentence constituent (i.e., either the argument or adjunct phrase) and replace it with the proper wh-morpheme, (c) identify the thematic roles of NPs in their new sentence positions, and (d) produce the surface form of targeted wh-questions. See Thompson (1996) for additional detail.

B. Training *Wh-* and NP-Movement Structures

1. Stimuli

Wh-movement structures: who-questions and object clefts ($N = 30$)
1. Who-question. *Who has the biker lifted?*
2. Object cleft. *It was the student who the biker lifted.*
   NP-movement structures: passives and subject raising (N = 30)
3. Passive. *The student was lifted by the biker.*
4. Subject-raising. *The biker seems to have lifted the student.*

2. Baseline and Treatment Probe Procedure.
Target sentences were tested using the sentence production priming task. This task entailed (a) presentation of a semantically reversible picture pair, (b) modeling the target sentence type with one picture from the pair, and (c) instructing JD to produce a similar sentence using the other picture. A 10-second response time was allowed.

3. **Treatment Procedures.** Using the active form of target sentences, the examiner identified the verb while pointing to it. For example, when training object clefts such as, *It was the artist who the thief chased,* the active form, [the thief] [chased] [the artist] was used. The examiner explained: "The action in this picture is *chased.* Someone chased someone." The subject and object NPs were identified and their roles in relation to the verb were explained. The *who* card then was placed next to the object NP and the examiner explained: "The thief is the person doing the chasing and the artist is the person *who* was chased." The object NP and *who* cards were then moved to the sentence initial position and the examiner explained: "We're going to make a new sentence about the thief and the artist. To do this *the artist* and *who* move to the beginning." The *it was* card then was placed at the beginning of the sentence while the examiner explained: "To make the new sentence, *It was* is added to the beginning." JD then was instructed to read the new sentence. Finally, the sentence constituent cards were rearranged in their original order and JD was instructed to move the cards to form the target sentence. JD then produced the derived noncanonical sentence and identified the thematic roles of NPs in their new positions. Assistance was provided as needed. The foil picture stimulus then was re-presented and the sentence production priming procedure was repeated. (See Thompson (1996) for training steps for each sentence type.)

CHAPTER

7

Treatment for Letter-by-Letter Reading: A Case Study

PELAGIE M. BEESON, Ph.D.

I. LETTER-BY-LETTER READING

Literate adults typically read familiar words in a holistic manner. They rarely need to identify individual letters explicitly because the entire word form is easily recognized as a single unit. When whole-word recognition is selectively impaired due to brain damage, however, sequential letter identification may be required in order to read. This letter-by-letter reading strategy is often observed in individuals with alexia without agraphia, also known as pure alexia. Such individuals capture clinical attention because of their surprising difficulty reading what they themselves have just written or by their overt spelling aloud of words as they try to read. Patterson and Kay (1982) described a patient with this syndrome: "he identifies each letter of the word in succession, often but not invariably naming the letter aloud as it is identified; when he has reached the end (or nearly the end) of the sequence of letters, he produces the word" (p. 413). Thus, letter-by-letter reading can be a useful compensatory strategy for pure alexia, but it typically results in a painstakingly slow reading rate that may warrant therapy.

A. Historical Perspective

Over a century ago, Déjerine (1891, 1892) described two patients with acquired reading impairments associated with lesions in the left hemisphere. One patient had a lesion involving the left parietal lobe resulting in alexia and agraphia. A second patient had a lesion of the left occipital lobe and splenium of the corpus callosum that produced alexia without agraphia. Based on these cases, Déjerine hypothesized that alexia with agraphia represented a destruction of the center for visual memory of words, which he localized to the left angular gyrus. In contrast, he hypothesized that alexia without agraphia represented a disconnection between the visual input and word forms in the left angular gyrus. A schematic drawing of such a lesion is shown in Figure 7–1; it includes damage to the visual cortex of the left occipital lobe (affecting the right visual field) and damage to the corpus callosum that disrupts transmission of visual information from the right hemisphere (i.e., the left visual field). As a result, the visual input fails to reach the left angular gyrus for word-form identification.

Déjerine's patient with alexia without agraphia reportedly could not identify letters and, therefore, had no alternative reading strategy. However, some individuals with pure alexia are able to identify letters with reasonable success and employ a strategy of word identification that results from sequential identification of the component letters of a word—that is, letter-by-letter reading (Patterson & Kay, 1982; Rapcsak, Rubens, & Laguna, 1990).

B. A Cognitive Processing Model of Reading

Figure 7–2 depicts letter-by-letter reading from an information processing perspective (see also Patterson & Kay, 1982; Rapcsak et al., 1990). The retinotopic representation of written text is transformed to a sequence of abstract letter identities that are independent of font or handwriting features. In the normal reading process, the visual letter-form analysis system provides access to the abstract visual word form (also referred to as the orthographic input lexicon), which activates the semantic representation of the word. A disconnection of the letter-form analysis system and word-form system (path a) results in failed recogni-

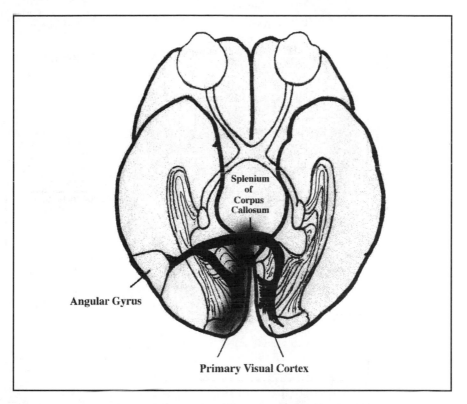

Figure 7–1. Schematic drawing of the efferent pathways critical for reading with a superimposed lesion in the left visual cortex and the splenium of the corpus callosum that would result in alexia without agraphia. The lesion is indicated by dark shading.

tion of a word that is visually perceived. Letter-by-letter reading is accomplished by an alternate processing route whereby individual letters are named (via path b) and serially transmitted to the word-form system (via path c).

The model presented here is consistent with that of Patterson and Kay (1982), but differs from that proposed by Warrington and Shallice (1980), who suggested that the word-form system, itself, is impaired in such cases. Other researchers have suggested that pure alexia is simply the most obvious manifestation of a more general visual impairment that slows or disrupts the ability to recognize complex visual stimuli (Farah & Wallace, 1991; Friedman & Alexander, 1984). These researchers proposed that reading is impaired because whole words are too visually

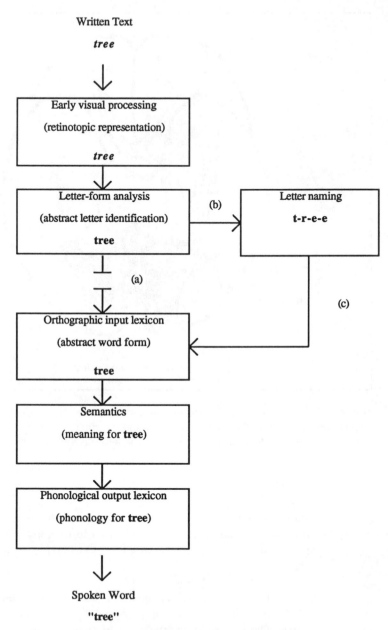

Figure 7–2. Model of letter-by-letter reading after Patterson and Kay (1982) and Rapcsak, Rubens, and Laguna (1990). The disconnection of the letter-form analysis system and the orthographic input lexicon (path a) is compensated for by letter-by-letter reading via paths b and c.

complex to be recognized, and the letter-by-letter reading strategy is adopted to compensate for this visual impairment.

The precise nature of the processing impairment in alexia without agraphia and the letter-by-letter reading strategy remains to be clarified. Better understanding of the underlying deficit should help guide the development of treatment approaches. At the same time, however, treatment studies should also contribute to our understanding of the reading impairment and normal reading processes (Behrmann & McLeod, 1995). The goal of this case report is twofold: to increase understanding about reading and pure alexia and to describe a useful treatment approach for letter-by-letter reading.

C. Common Clinical Features of Letter-by-Letter Readers

1. **The characteristic features of letter-by-letter reading include:**

    a. **Word recognition** accomplished by means of **sequential letter identification,** either aloud or subvocally.

    b. **Word length effect**
        (1) **Slow reading rate** that is related to word length (i.e., increasingly slower as word length increases).
        (2) **Reading accuracy decreases** as a function of word length.

    c. **No effects of lexical features**
        (1) **No advantage for high frequency** words over low frequency words.
        (2) **No advantage of high imagery** (i.e., concrete) over low imagery (i.e., abstract) words.
        (3) **No advantage for part of speech** (nouns versus verbs and adjectives versus functors)

    d. **No effects of regularity of spelling** so that words that have good sound-to-letter correspondence are not notably easier than irregularly spelled words.

2. **Common impairments associated with letter-by-letter reading include:**

    a. **Letter identification deficits,** for example, visually similar letters may be confused, e.g., p/b, r/f, m/w leading to such errors as "b-r-i-d-e, bride" for *pride*.

      b. Right homonymous hemianopia.

      c. Color naming deficits.

      d. Mild-to-moderate word-finding difficulties.

  3. Unaffected processes typically include:

      a. Intact speech production and writing ability.

      b. Relatively intact number reading.

D. Neurological Findings

Letter-by-letter reading has been associated with lesions in the following locations:

  1. Left occipital lobe and splenium of the corpus callosum. This is the classic alexia without agraphia profile (Déjerine, 1892) shown in Figure 7–1.

  2. White matter lesion isolating the left angular gyrus, sometimes called subangular alexia without agraphia (Greenblatt, 1976) because the lesion is deep to the angular gyrus.

  3. Other cortical or subcortical lesions that preserve the integrity of the angular gyrus but block visual input to the angular gyrus (Damasio & Damasio, 1983) including:

      a. Left lateral occipital damage.

      b. Unilateral left occipitoparietal, temporal, or temporo-parietal lesion.

II. CASE REPORT OF A LETTER-BY-LETTER READER

A. Biography

HL was a right-handed, English-speaking male with 11 years of formal education. He had a history of steady employment as an industrial plumber with an aeronautics firm. Prior to his stroke, he reported reading trade magazines on a regular basis and also enjoyed reading adventure/spy novels for pleasure. HL's writing was essentially restricted to notes and lists of things to buy or do. He reported that numerous spelling errors were common ever since childhood.

B. Medical History

1. **Acute event.** HL had a relatively unremarkable medical history, with the exception of hypertension, recently diagnosed borderline diabetes, and mild obesity. At age 53, he experienced an abrupt onset of headache behind his left eye and blurred vision. He recalled answering the phone at his home, writing down a message, and then realizing shortly thereafter that he could not read his own writing. HL initially contacted his ophthalmologist and was admitted to the hospital that day for more comprehensive evaluation.

2. **Initial examination**

   a. **Initial neurological examination** during hospitalization showed that HL was alert and oriented with no evidence of aphasia, dysarthria, or apraxia. A motor examination was normal for strength, tone, and fine motor movements. His sensory examination was also normal, but a visual field defect was suspected. He had marked difficulty with reading, although he was able to write.

   b. **CT head scan** showed a hemorrhagic infarction in the territory of the left posterior cerebral artery affecting the left posterior occipito-temporal region extending into subjacent white matter (Figure 7–3).

3. **Visual examination.** Formal, automated visual field testing at 4 days poststroke showed an incongruous right hemianopia of greater density in the superior quadrant (Figure 7–4). At 5 weeks poststroke, however, repeated visual field testing documented nearly complete resolution of the visual field defect.

C. Initial Speech-Language Evaluation

At 2 weeks poststroke, HL's speech-language pathologist administered subtests from the *Minnesota Test for Differential Diagnosis of Aphasia* (MTDDA; Schuell, 1972), the *Boston Naming Test* (BNT; Kaplan, Goodglass, & Weintraub, 1983), and the *Reading Comprehension Battery for Adults* (RCBA; LaPointe & Horner, 1979).

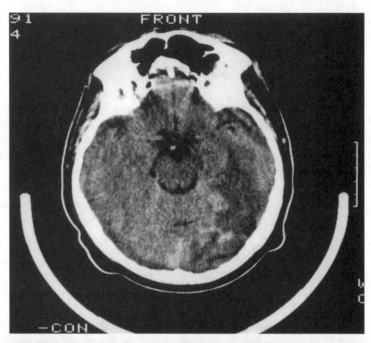

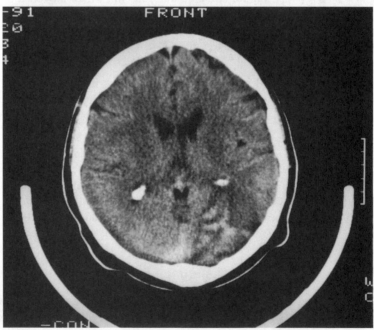

Figure 7–3. Acute CT head scan of patient HL showing a hemorrhagic infarction in the left posterior occipito-temporal region

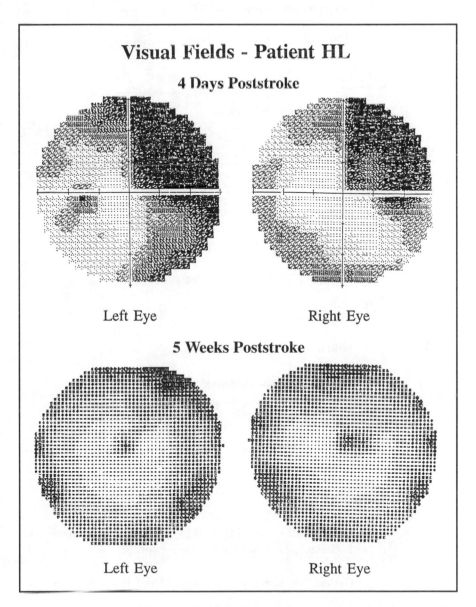

Figure 7–4. Results of HL's visual field testing at 4 days and 5 weeks poststroke. The initial examination revealed a right hemianopia of greater density in the superior quadrant (dark shading). The second examination showed nearly complete resolution of the defect.

1. Auditory comprehension (MTDDA)

   a. Sentences   100%

   b. Paragraphs   100%

2. Verbal expression (MTDDA)

   a. Sentence repetition   100%

   b. Producing sentences   84%

   c. Picture description   100%

   d. Defining words   90%

   e. Retelling a paragraph   84%

3. Writing (MTDDA)

   a. Written spelling of single words   60%

   b. Producing written sentences   67%

   c. Writing a paragraph   50%

Writing included numerous spelling errors. Sentences and paragraph description lacked some functors.

4. Naming

   a. Confrontation naming (BNT) 52/60—slightly more than 1 standard deviation below the mean for age.

   b. Generative naming (animals) 18/minute—within normal limits.

5. Reading (RCBA)

   a. Single-word match-to-pictures—27/30 = 90% correct with an extremely slow reading rate of 9 seconds/word = 6.6 words per minute. Overt letter-by-letter reading was observed.

    b. Sentence and paragraph reading—no words were identified and testing was discontinued.

6. **Summary of language abilities at 2 weeks postonset.** Auditory comprehension and verbal expression were roughly within normal limits, except for confrontation naming, which appeared to be mildly impaired. HL was not able to read sentence- or paragraph-level text. Single-word reading was accomplished by letter-by-letter reading that was extremely slow, but fairly accurate. Written spelling and discourse were considered below average.

III. APPRAISAL

At 6 weeks poststroke, HL was referred to me by his speech-language pathologist for further assessment and treatment of his reading impairment.

A. Rationale and Method

The goal of the evaluation was to characterize the nature of the reading problem and rule out concomitant impairments.

1. **Patient description.** HL provided a useful description of his problem and use of a letter-by-letter reading strategy.

   Well, I just don't read. One word at a time, I can pick it out if I work at it. Like, different things like directions or a street sign. If I look at a street sign long enough, I'll get it. I have to spell things . . . and sometimes I have to put my finger and block out a long word, so that I take the word apart and figure it out that way. I have to do that.

2. **Reading performance** was assessed to confirm the presence of the primary clinical features of letter-by-letter reading.

       a. Single-word reading was tested to look for effects of word length on reading accuracy and to determine if reading was influenced by lexical features such as frequency, imagery, or word-class.

       b. Individual letter identification was tested.

       c. Reading rate and comprehension of text were assessed.

3. **Writing** and other relevant domains were assessed.

B. Results

1. **Single word reading.** Controlled lists of 140 words from the *Battery of Adult Reading Function* (Rothi, Coslett, & Heilman, 1984) were presented for reading aloud with no time constraints. Testing was accomplished over 4 sessions between 6 and 8 weeks poststroke. The following lexical variables were examined.

   a. **Word frequency.** Reading accuracy was not better for high frequency words compared to low frequency words.

   High frequency = 20/40 = 50%

   Low frequency = 29/40 = 72%

   b. **Imagery.** Reading accuracy was not better for high imagery words compared to low imagery words.

   High imagery = 21/40 = 52%

   Low imagery = 28/40 = 70%

   c. **Part of speech.** No effects.

   Nouns = 90/140 = 64%

   Verbs = 14/20 = 70%

   Functors = 14/20 = 70%

   Prefixed, suffixed, derivational = 15/24 = 62%

   d. **Able to read pronounceable nonwords** with fair accuracy

   Nonwords = 14/20 = 70%

   e. **Regularity of spelling** did not affect spelling accuracy.

   Regular spelling = 32/60 = 53%

   Irregular spelling = 38/60 = 63%

   f. **Word length effect** for reading accuracy was not linear, but accuracy was notably reduced for seven-letter words compared with shorter words. (Reaction times for single-word reading were not obtained until 6 months postonset, at which time the software for computer presentation was obtained. See section VII.C.)

4 Letters = 71%

5 Letters = 80%

6 Letters = 77%

7 Letters = 42%

g. **In summary.** There were no significant effects of word frequency, imagery, or part of speech. Nonwords were read with accuracy similar to real words, thus indicating an ability to sound-out words. Regularly spelled words were not read more accurately than irregular words, indicating that there was not an overreliance on letter-to-sound correspondences. The most notable characteristics of HL's reading were his extremely slow reading rate for all types of words and his occasional overt letter-by-letter reading. Error frequency was notably greater for 7-letter words compared with 4-, 5-, and 6 letter words.

2. Letter naming

a. No errors occurred in naming individual letters; however, letter identification errors were made when reading letters of single words.

b. No errors occurred in producing sounds associated with vowels and consonants of the English alphabet, such as "p" makes the sound "puh."

3. **Text reading.** Levels 1 through 6 of the *Gray Oral Reading Test—Revised* (GORT-R; Wiederholt & Bryant, 1986)—Form A was administered to assess text reading rate and comprehension. At 10 weeks postonset of stroke, HL's reading rates were considerably slower than typical adult oral reading rates of 150 to 200 words per minute (wpm; Rayner & Pollatsek, 1989).

Level 1	14 wpm	Level 5	13 wpm
Level 2	11 wpm	Level 6	12 wpm
Level 3	9 wpm	Mean =	12.5 wpm
Level 4	16 wpm		

HL's reading comprehension was not impaired. He responded correctly to 80 to 100% of questions on the GORT-R passages.

4. Writing. Most errors were phonologically plausible spellings, although there was not a consistent pattern of phonological spelling in that some irregularly spelled words (e.g., knife) were correct. HL asserted that his writing abilities had not changed as a result of the stroke; samples of his premorbid writing were obtained and confirmed his assertion.

5. Other domains

a. **Number reading** was unimpaired. Some calculation errors were observed with simple mental calculation and written calculation for 3- and 4-digit numbers. HL indicated that these problems were consistent with his premorbid mathematical ability.

b. **Color naming** was not impaired.

c. **Normal visual memory for faces** as measured by the *Recognition Memory Test for Faces* (Warrington, 1984) was 48/50 correct = 93.5%ile.

IV. DIAGNOSIS

HL displayed the clinical syndrome of pure alexia; more specifically, he was a letter-by-letter reader. This disorder existed in the relative absence of other acquired neuropsychological deficits. Spoken and written communication, auditory comprehension, color identification, visual processing and memory for faces, number identification, and calculation all appeared commensurate with premorbid abilities. HL was somewhat unusual in that his premorbid writing contained many spelling errors, but there was no evidence of acquired impairment of writing due to his stroke.

V. PROGNOSIS

A. Prognostic Signs

HL was motivated to work on his reading in the hope that he could return to work and again be able to read for pleasure. His relatively good letter recognition and the absence of significant concomitant language or cognitive problems were positive prognostic signs for reading improvement.

B. Expected Outcome

Improved reading rate with preserved comprehension was the expected treatment outcome.

VI. FOCUSING THE TREATMENT

A. Rationale

1. **The treatment goal** was to facilitate text reading and increase reading rate, maintaining accuracy and comprehension to the extent that it was functional for basic needs, work, and personal enjoyment.

2. **Treatment literature.** Limited literature exists regarding therapy for letter-by-letter readers. A therapy program described by Moyer (1979), however, provided evidence of increased reading rate in a person with acquired alexia who appeared to be a letter-by-letter reader secondary to an embolic occipital infarct. Moyers designed a program that entailed repeated oral readings of written passages that resulted in improved reading rate for previously unread material. Moody (1988a) and Tuomainen and Laine (1991) also reported case studies supporting a multiple oral reading (MOR) approach for letter-by-letter readers.

   Some treatments for pure alexia have been directed toward the single-word level rather than connected text. Moody (1988b) showed improved reading accuracy for affixed words that were treated in isolation rather than text. Rothi and Moss (1992) used rapid computer presentation of single words to facilitate a shift from letter-by-letter reading to direct access to word meaning. The treatment was successful in one patient (Rothi & Moss, 1992), but the positive effects were not replicated in a subsequent case (Rothi, Greenwald, Maher, & Ochipa, Chapter 8). Behrmann and McLeod (1995) also attempted to facilitate parallel, rather than serial, processing of letters in single words with a treatment task that required rapid identification of first and last letters of words presented on a computer screen. Their treatment was successful in improving recognition of the right-most letters in single words presented at increasingly rapid rates; however, the treatment did not facilitate a change in single-word reading performance in that the word-length effect persisted.

3. **Text reading** was selected as the target of treatment rather than single-word reading, because the semantic and syntactic structure

of text offered contextual information to assist in word identification. Text reading was also considered a more ecologically valid activity than reading word lists, and improved reading for text was the desired outcome for HL.

4. **Hypothesis.** Repeated reading of the same text should facilitate whole-word reading because of the increased familiarity with a passage. It was hypothesized that improved word recognition in the context of familiar text would serve to facilitate direct access to word forms when reading new text. Therefore, improved whole-word recognition should reduce (or eliminate) the use of the letter-by-letter reading strategy and should increase reading rate.

B. Methods

1. **Therapy materials.** Because they are controlled for length and complexity, passages from the *Scientific Research Associates Reading Laboratory* (SRA, 1978) were selected as stimuli. The passages from grade levels 2.5 to 6.0 were used. They ranged in length from 250 to 700 words, with incremental increase in sentence complexity and mean word length. The content of the SRA reading passages was considered to be of high interest and fairly appropriate for an adult reader.

C. Procedure

a. **Baseline reading rates** were obtained on three SRA stories (grade level 2.5) over 3 weeks (from 8 weeks to 10 weeks postonset).

b. **During a six-month period,** hour-long therapy sessions were scheduled twice-a-week for the first 5 months and once-a-week for the last month of therapy. Some sessions were canceled because of vacations and other appointments, resulting in a total of 30 treatment sessions.

c. **Therapy** consisted of repeatedly reading target passages aloud with the goal of increased reading rate and accuracy. Reading errors were pointed out for self-correction or were corrected by the clinician when self-correction failed. Reading rates were calculated and plotted over time with the target goal of 100 wpm for the practiced (i.e., re-read) passages. When that goal was reached for a given passage, a new passage was introduced for initial reading rate assessment and then repeated reading.

d. Homework was a critical component of treatment; HL was instructed to read designated passages aloud at least three times daily. He kept a daily log to indicate each re-reading. HL typically read two SRA passages each three times per day.

D. Outcome Measures

1. Reading rates for SRA texts were obtained each time a new text was introduced for the re-reading task. Those rates were plotted to determine if the treatment was influencing reading rate for new material.

2. The *Gray Oral Reading Test–Revised* (GORT-R; Wiederholt & Bryant, 1986). Form B, Levels 1 through 6 were administered as post-test measures of reading rate and comprehension.

VII. RESULTS

A. Reading Rate for Practiced Text

HL successfully achieved a reading rate of 100 wpm for 13 SRA passages that were repeatedly practiced. Figure 7–5 shows the typical improvement in reading rate over time for 4 of the passages that were ultimately read at 100 wpm.

B. Reading Rate for New Text

1. **Reading rates** for previously unread SRA texts are displayed in Figure 7–6. Baseline reading rates were stable over 4 weeks, averaging 11 words per minute (i.e., about 5.5 seconds per word) for reading passages at 2.5 grade level. Following the initiation of treatment, HL showed relatively steady improvement in reading rate and higher-level passages were introduced as indicated in Figure 7–6. A notable drop in reading rate was observed as SRA levels 5 and then 6 were introduced, which prompted a return to levels 2.5 to 3.5 to monitor rate. At the end of 6 months, reading rates were averaging about 35 wpm (i.e., about 1.7 seconds per word) for SRA level 3.0.

2. **Figure 7–7 shows the change in reading rate** on the GORT-R from the initiation of therapy (10 weeks postonset of stroke) and after 6 months of treatment (10 months postonset of stroke).

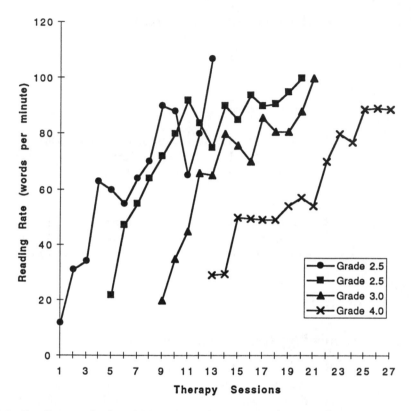

Figure 7–5. Reading rate for four SRA passages that were read repeatedly to increase reading rate to 100 w.p.m. Performance on these passages was representative of improved rate on other passages that were practiced repeatedly as homework.

Pretreatment = Average of levels 1–6 = 12.5 wpm (maximum = 16 wpm)

Posttreatment = Average of levels 1–6 = 28 wpm (maximum = 40 wpm)

Reading rate increased by more than 100% after 6 months of treatment.

3. **Although HL's oral reading rate was still far below normal** (150–200 wpm) at the end of treatment, the improvement provided a reading ability that permitted him to read newspaper, mail, and work-related instructions. HL also reported a return to some pleasure reading. Unfortunately HL was not allowed to return to work

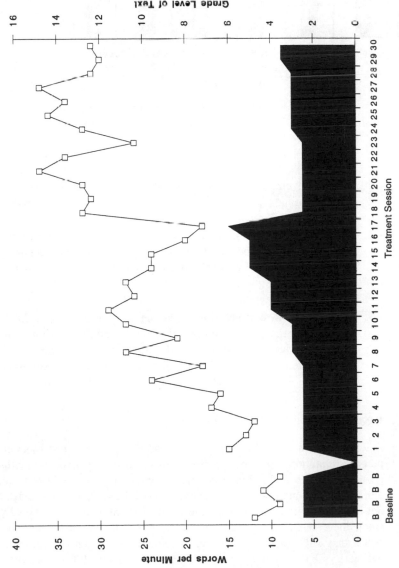

Figure 7–6. Reading rate for SRA passages that were new to HL. Baseline measures were taken over 4 weeks before initiation of the MOR treatment. The grade level of the text is indicated by the dark shading and is marked on the right ordinate

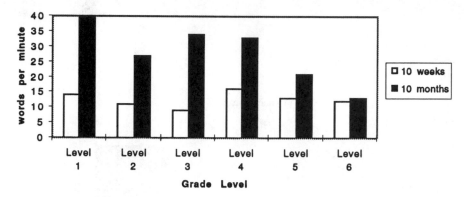

Figure 7–7. Reading rates for HL on the GORT-R before and after treatment to increase reading rate. The difficulty of the reading passage increases from Level 1 to 6.

because of employer concerns about his health and the physical demands of his job.

4. **HL's reading comprehension remained high** throughout the treatment period. He responded to questions with 80 to 100% accuracy on the GORT-R, and was able to summarize reading passages with considerable accuracy.

5. **Long-term follow-up testing** of reading rate was performed almost 2 years after the termination of treatment. Re-administration of the GORT-R (Form A) showed that HL had continued to improve his reading rate after the termination of therapy. Two-year Follow-up = Average of levels 1–6 = 69 wpm (maximum = 100 wpm)

C. Reading Rate for Single Words

Precise reaction times for single-word reading were obtained by computer presentation at 6 months postonset of stroke and again at 10 months postonset (Figure 7–8). Reaction times were measured from the time the word appeared on the screen to the initiation of the spoken word, and did not include the time taken to say the word. Normal readers show a very small increase in reading time as word length increases (Henderson, 1982; Just & Carpenter, 1980), but a marked word-length effect is the hallmark of letter-by-letter reading (Patterson & Kay, 1982). The correlation between word length and HL's reaction time was significant at 6 months ($r = 0.979$) and 10 months ($r = 0.965$) postonset indicating a marked word-length effect on both occasions. The persistence of the

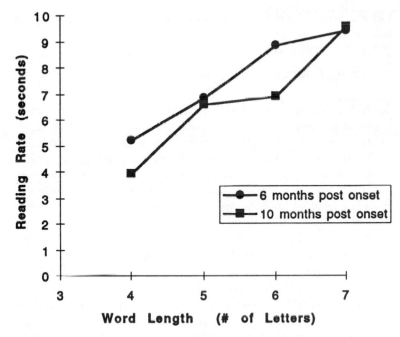

Figure 7–8. Reaction times for reading 4-, 5-, 6-, and 7-letter words presented individually on a computer screen.

word-length effect was surprising because HL's text reading at 10 months poststroke did not give the impression of a letter-by-letter strategy, and there were few instances of overt letter-by-letter reading. It was also noteworthy that HL's reading rate for single words did not significantly improve from 6 to 10 months postonset ($t = 1.77$), although reading rate for text improved during that time. At 10 months postonset HL's reading rate for single words was considerably slower than reading words in text (about 6.7 seconds versus 1.7 seconds, respectively).

VIII. DISCUSSION

HL improved his reading rate for text over the 6 months of treatment while maintaining a high level of comprehension. At the beginning of therapy, at 10 weeks poststroke, he reported that he was essentially not reading text (other than in test situations). After treatment, his reading rate was sufficient to allow him to read as needed for everyday tasks and even to read for pleasure. Two questions are worthy of discussion: (1) Was the improvement due to treatment or did it reflect the natural recovery process? (2) What was the mechanism whereby HL's reading improved?

A. Treatment Effect versus Spontaneous Recovery

1. **HL's reading rate for text was stable** for 4 weeks prior to treatment as reflected by the four baseline measures for SRA passages. Over the 6 months of treatment, his reading rate for new text steadily increased. This slow, consistent recovery extending beyond 6 months postonset was not characteristic of spontaneous recovery curves which are steepest during the first 3 months poststroke and show relatively little change after 6 months postonset (Kertesz, 1997). The fact that single-word reading rate remained stable from 6 to 10 months postonset, with text reading rate increasing during that time, suggests that there was a specific treatment effect for text versus single-word reading.

2. **That HL's reading rate for text continued to improve** after the termination of treatment could be interpreted as evidence of natural recovery; however, it is also plausible that treatment enabled HL to return to text reading, and his independent reading continued to have a rehabilitative effect.

3. **In conclusion,** HL's improvement was more suggestive of a positive treatment effect than spontaneous recovery, but the contribution of natural recovery cannot be ruled out completely and additional treatment cases are needed to clarify the effects of treatment versus natural recovery.

B. Mechanism of Recovery

1. **Treatment** was intended to facilitate whole-word reading, and thus reduce the need for letter-by-letter reading. HL's reading rate of 100 wpm for practiced text was clearly too fast to reflect a letter-by-letter approach and appeared to demonstrate a return to whole-word reading in that supported context. His oral reading of new text also lost the outward appearance of a letter-by-letter strategy; but it remained slow enough so that some covert letter-by-letter reading was probably still used at 10 months postonset, in combination with whole-word recognition. It was noteworthy that HL continued to improve his reading rate in the year following therapy and achieved rates up to 100 wpm for new text, suggesting that

direct access to the visual word-form system was re-established, to some extent.

2. **The treatment effect was relatively selective for text reading.** Single-word reading times measured via computer presentation were dramatically slower than text reading and single-word reading retained a marked word-length effect, suggesting persistence of letter-by-letter reading in that context. The improved rate for text reading suggested that HL was taking advantage of semantic and syntactic information to assist in word recognition when reading passages. He may have improved his ability to use a top-down strategy whereby contextual information was coupled with identification of the initial letters of a word to facilitate word recognition, obviating the need for serial identification of each letter. Alternatively, HL's direct whole-word recognition may have improved to the extent that it was functional when supported by context.

3. **The MOR treatment facilitated increased reading rate,** however, the dissociation of text and single-word reading may indicate that HL did not achieve a return to normal reading processes. His direct access to word forms (path a in Figure 7–2) did not appear to be fully operational, yet there was evidence that he was not fully dependent upon the alternate letter-by-letter route (path b to c). His improvement may have reflected a summation of improved direct access to word forms in some contexts (path a) and interactive processing of serial letter identification and whole-word recognition.

C. Hindsight

HL was seen twice a week for most of the 6 months of treatment. In retrospect, the program may have been accomplished with less frequent or fewer sessions, because the sessions were primarily directed toward monitoring the home program. Weekly sessions may have been sufficient so long as daily homework was completed.

IX. SUMMARY

This clinical case offers support for the multiple oral reading approach for the treatment of letter-by-letter reading. It is a relatively simple clinical procedure that depends largely on patient motivation to work on reading at home. Therefore, it may be an effective treatment approach when reimbursement dollars are limited. Further research is needed for complete understanding of the rehabilitative effect of this approach and to characterize the best candidates.

X. ACKNOWLEDGMENT

I thank Thomas Slauson, CCC-SLP for his referral and clinical assistance with this patient. This work was supported, in part, by National Multipurpose Research and Training Center Grant DC-01409 from the National Institute on Deafness and Other Communication Disorders.

XI. REFERENCES

Behrmann, M., & McLeod, J. (1995). Rehabilitation for pure alexia: Efficacy of therapy and implications for models of normal word recognition. *Neuropsychological rehabilitation, 5,* 149–180.

Damasio, A. R., & Damasio, H. (1983). The anatomic basis of pure alexia. *Neurology, 33,* 1573–1583.

Déjerine, J. (1891). Sur en case de cecite verbal avec agraphie, suivi d'autopsie. *Compete Rendu Hebdomadaire des Sceances et Memoires de la Societe de Biologie, 3,* 197–201.

Déjerine, J. (1892). Contribution a l'etude anatomo-pathologique et clinique des differentes varietes de cecite verbale. *Compete Rendu Hebdomadaire des Sceances et Memoires de la Societe de Biologie, 4,* 61–90.

Farah, M. J., & Wallace, M. A. (1991). Pure alexia as a visual impairment: A reconsideration. *Cognitive neuropsychology, 8,* 313–334.

Friedman, R. B., & Alexander, M. P. (1984). Pictures, images and pure alexia: A case study. *Cognitive neuropsychology, 1,* 9–23.

Greenblatt, S. H. (1976). Subangular alexia without agraphia or hemianopsia. *Brain and Language, 3,* 229–245.

Henderson, L. (1982). *Orthography and word recognition in reading.* London: Academic Press.

Just, M. A., & Carpenter, P. A. (1980). The theory of reading: From eye fixations to comprehension. *Psychological Review, 87,* 329–354.

Kaplan, E., Goodglass, H., & Weintraub, S. (1983). *The Boston Naming Test.* Philadelphia: Lea & Febiger.

Kertesz, A. (1997). Recovery of aphasia. In T. E. Feinberg & M. J. Farah (Eds.), *Behavioral neurology and neuropsychology,* pp. 167–182. New York: McGraw-Hill.

LaPointe, L., & Horner, J. (1979). *Reading Comprehension Battery for Adults.* Tigard, OR: CC Publications.

Moody, S. (1988a). The Moyer reading technique re-evaluated. *Cortex, 24,* 474–476.

Moody, S. (1988b). Rehabilitation of acquired dyslexia. *Clinical Rehabilitation, 2,* 291–298.

Moyer, S. B. (1979). Rehabilitation of alexia: A case study. *Cortex, 15,* 139–144.

Patterson, K., & Kay, K. (1982). Letter-by-letter reading: Psychological descriptions of a neurological description of a neurological syndrome. *Quarterly Journal of Experimental Psychology, 34A,* 411–441.

Rapcsak, S. Z., Rubens, A. B., & Laguna, J. F. (1990). From letters to words: Procedures for word recognition in letter-by-letter reading. *Brain and Language, 38,* 504–514.

Rayner, R., & Pollatsek, A. (1989). *The psychology of reading.* Englewood Cliffs, NJ: Prentice Hall.

Rothi, L. J., Coslett, H. B., & Heilman, K. M. (1984). *Battery of adult reading function,* Experimental edition. Unpublished.

Rothi, L. J. G., & Moss, S. (1992). Alexia without agraphia: Potential for model assisted therapy. *Clinics in communication disorders, 2,* 11–18.

Schuell, H. (1972). *The Minnesota Test for Differential Diagnosis of Aphasia.* Minneapolis: University of Minnesota Press.

SRA Reading Laboratory, Mark II Series (1978). Scientific Research Associates, Inc. Don H. Parker, Director, Institute for Multilevel Learning International Incorporated.

Tuomainen, J., & Laine, M. (1991). *Aphasiology, 5,* 401–409.

Wiederholt, J. L. & Bryant, B. P. (1986) *Gray Oral Reading Test–Revised,* Austin, TX: PRO-ED.

Warrington, E. K. (1984). *Recognition Memory Test for Faces.* Los Angeles: Western Psychological Services.

Warrington, E. K., & Shallice, T. (1980). Word-form dyslexia. *Brain, 103,* 99–112.

CHAPTER

8

Alexia Without Agraphia:
Lessons From a Treatment Failure

LESLIE J. GONZALEZ ROTHI, PH.D.
MARGARET L. GREENWALD, PH.D.
LYNN M. MAHER, PH.D.
CYNTHIA OCHIPA, PH.D.

I. BACKGROUND

A. Functional System Underlying Reading and Pure Alexia

1. **Déjerine (1891, 1892) described two types of acquired reading disorders** that are anatomically and functionally distinctive.

    a. **Anatomic Differences**
      (1) **Alexia without agraphia (word blindness).** A lesion of the left occipital lobe, usually found in the lingual and fusiform gyri.

(2) **Alexia with agraphia.** Typically involves lesions associated with the left parietal lobe.

b. **Functional differences.** The functional mechanisms of these disorders differ, implying that the treatments should be different as well.

(1) **Alexia without agraphia.** Although Déjerine posited that occipital lesions disconnect visual input from visual word forms stored in the left parietal lobe, others proposed that pure alexia is induced by a perceptual deficit.

(2) **Alexia with agraphia.** This is a disorder that results from deficits involving lexical (word-recognition/word-meaning) components utilized by both the reading and written spelling systems.

Because we report on a treatment of a case of alexia without agraphia, the remainder of this paper focuses on the mechanism of pure alexia only.

2. **The perceptual system supporting reading;** a system utilizing both hemispheres.

a. **The left occipital lobe** provides rapid, parallel visual processing of letters in words that:

(1) **Have "privileged" access** to the lexicon (word recognition system) (Figure 8–1, a) (Ellis, Young, & Anderson, 1988); and

(2) **This "privileged processor"** is insensitive to letter form in that it is not influenced by physical alterations such as changes in font or letter size.

b. **Both hemispheres have a second processor** of seen words available that we call the "segmental processor" (Figure 8–1, b) which is:

(1) **Influenced by word length,**

(2) **Used when one processes unfamiliar words** and words printed in abnormal fonts, and

(3) **Is thought to process seen words** with letters in initial and final positions of words processed first, followed by more medially placed letters.

c. **In the case of alexia without agraphia** from a left occipital lesion:

(1) **The privileged processor** is impaired and does not have "privileged access" to the lexicon, but

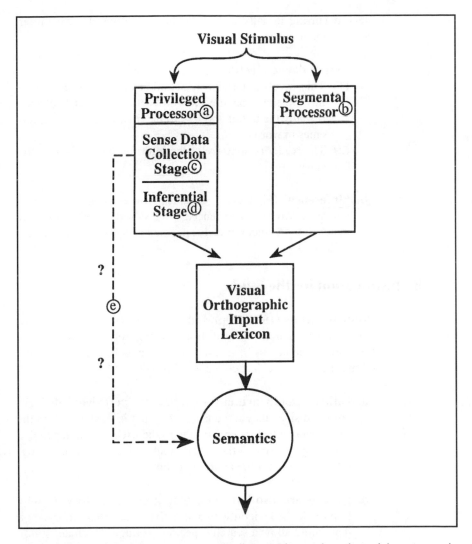

Figure 8–1. Model of the process involved in single-word reading elaborating early visual analysis

    (2) The segmental processor may remain functional and the patient may be left to read only with the assistance of this processor using a segmental style of visual word processing; reading effortfully and slowly, one letter at a time.

3. The privileged processor has two stages (Henderson, 1987) that are necessarily temporally related, with the "sense data collection"

stage occurring initially and for a short duration and the "inference" stage occurring subsequently.

    a. "Sense data collection" (Figure 8–1, c).

        (1) This involves passive registration of sensory data in an incompletely specified array of letters and letter clusters (usually the initial and less so the final positions of graphemes in words).

        (2) The reader is unaware of the information obtained in this stage.

    b. "Inference" (Figure 8–1, d). This involves a matching process where previously experienced (and stored) letter strings are matched to the incompletely specified array of the "sense data collection."

B. Justification for the Study

1. Rothi and Moss (1992) reported a case in which alexia without agraphia was thought to result from an "inference" deficit within the "privileged access" system of word recognition in the context of sparing of "sense data collection." In this condition:

    a. Patients would be unaware of having "perceived" the written word since they are unaware of what is "collected" in the sense data collector. This results in their feeling unprepared at later stages to search the visual input lexicon (the word recognition system) for the appropriate lexeme.

    b. Patients are also left to develop a compensatory strategy to provide the lexicon with alternative but explicit information that would allow a search (Speedie, Rothi, & Heilman, 1982). In the case of letter-by-letter readers, reading may rely exclusively on the segmental processor to access the lexicon, using a strategy that decomposes the seen word into its constituent parts.

2. If the compensating reader is limited to this inefficient letter-by-letter reading strategy, how might we develop a more productive reading strategy? If some pure alexia patients have normal "sense data collection," is the information available to the "sense data collector" capable of being utilized? Some patients with pure alexia of the letter-by-letter type can achieve at least some amount of semantic information for rapidly presented words they claim not to have "seen" (Bub, Black, & Behrmann, 1987; Coslett & Saffran, 1994; Shallice & Saffran, 1986). Thus, it is argued that the "sense data collector" has direct access to some minimal level of semantic information (Coslett & Saffran, 1994) (Figure 8–1, e). As the functional goal of reading is to extract meaning from seen words, it would seem important to help alexic patients to use this minimal amount of semantic information about words they are unaware of perceiving.

3. **A successful treatment program** to make alexic readers explicitly aware of the meanings of words they implicitly perceived was described by Rothi and Moss (1992). In this chapter, we report an attempt to replicate the efficacy of this approach in another pure alexia case.

II. THE PATIENT: MC

A. Biography

1. **A 72-year-old, right-handed, college educated man** who worked all his life in sales and then as a municipal financial director until retirement 4 years prior to his stroke.

2. Happily married with two sons living nearby.

3. Busy social life within small community.

4. No change in eating or sleeping habits.

5. No longer finds it enjoyable to read recreationally, because "it's effortful."

B. Medical History

1. **MC was in usual state of good health** until 13 months prior, when a sudden onset of "marked diminution of vision in the right eye" was noted. At that same time his wife reported "some change in his personality" with "mild confusion."

2. **Admission CT** reported to show "a rather large area of ill-defined, low density on the left that extended from above the tentorium into

the occipital lobe and extended caudally into the occipital-parietal junction."

3. **Admission neurologic exam** was notable for right homonymous hemianopsia, alexia without agraphia, and Gerstmann's syndrome (anomia, right/left disorientation, and finger anomia).

4. **Subsequent follow-up exams** revealed diminution in the severity of the alexia and anomia, lessening of his right visual field defect to a right superior quadrantanopia, with only a partial right inferior quadrantanopia and normalization of right/left orientation, digit span of six, written spelling, finger gnosis, praxis, and calculations. However MC was unable to remember three objects for 3 minutes and could name only the current president.

C. Previous Management

1. **MC was seen by a speech/language pathologist** from 49 days postonset until 4 months postonset.

2. **This therapy program** was reported to focus on a moderate difficulty "finding nouns," which was said to "resolve," and the patient was discharged as having received the maximum benefit of therapy.

III. APPRAISAL

A. Rationale

1. **We suspected that a direct route** (via the "sense data collector") to semantics that bypasses conscious awareness and explicit orthographic knowledge about seen words might be recruited to support/ circumvent a potentially deficient "word form" processor in MC.

2. **We knew that the patient** had a well-established diagnosis of alexia without agraphia and relatively little spoken language involvement with the exception of the "anomia" reported earlier. Therefore, our assessment goals were:

   a. **To document** the extent of his confrontation naming deficit,

   b. **To confirm** the presence of alexia and demonstrate relative sparing of written spelling, and

Table 8–1. *Western Aphasia Battery* (Kertesz, 1982)

Subtest	Possible	12 mpo
Spontaneous Speech	20	18
Information content	10	9
Fluency	10	9
Comprehension	10	9.65
Yes/No Questions	60	54
Auditory word Recognition	60	59
Sequential Commands	80	80
Repetition	10	9.7
Naming	10	6
Object Naming	60	26
Word Fluency	20	14
Sentence Completion	10	10
Responsive Speech	10	10
Aphasia Quotient	**100**	**86.7**
Reading	100	90
Writing	100	99
Praxis	60	60
Drawing	30	30
Calculation	24	24

c. **Because our therapy** would try to make implicit knowledge explicit, we needed to learn if MC was able to access implicit semantic information about seen words.

B. Methods and Results

All pretreatment testing was performed on consecutive days immediately preceding the initiation of treatment.

1. **Aphasia testing.** No speech or language impairments were noted except in confrontation naming.

a. *Western Aphasia Battery* (Kertesz, 1982). Aphasia quotient = 86.7 (see Table 8–1).

b. *Controlled Oral Word Association Test* (F, A, S, and semantic category) (norms reported by Spreen & Strauss, 1991). Mean score of 11.5 words in 60 seconds for words beginning with F, A, or S and 17.5 words in 60 seconds for words belonging to a semantic category (states or animals).

c. **Boston Naming Test,** BNT (Kaplan, Goodglass, & Weintraub, 1983). Total score of 26 correct/60 possible. Given semantic cues, MC responded with the target words 0/5 times versus 8/12 times when given phonemic cues. In 27 of the errors, MC gave semantic information relevant to the target. Seventeen of 26 correct responses were given during the first 30 of 60 items and involved higher frequency words.

d. **A modified version of the Boston Naming Test** (Kaplan et al., 1983), hereafter referred to as the *Boston Naming Test– Modified,* was administered, with exposure durations of the stimuli limited to 500 msec. This form of presentation was used to equalize the exposure durations of the printed material presented in this task to exposure durations in tasks such as the lexical decision task described in section III.B.3. We hoped to estimate if the problem found in MC's reading was found in other visual processing tasks that utilize nonorthographic stimuli (in this case, pictures of objects). When tested in this manner, MC's naming accuracy fell to 7 correct/60 possible. (*Response* durations on this and the BNT task described in the previous section were handled using the standard procedures of the instrument recommended by the authors.)

In summary, MC showed no apparent linguistic deficits except in visual confrontation naming. This deficit significantly worsened when the stimulus exposure was brief.

2. **Reading and spelling tests.** Tests given to assess reading and writing during the pretreatment sessions and results of MC's performances were:

a. **Schonell Test of Oral Word Reading** (Schonell, 1961). Word reading grade level = 13 years (of 15 years possible) (see Table 8–2).

b. **Reading aloud words varying in length.** If MC read by identifying each letter, then response latencies should be longer and risk of error should increase as the stimulus length increases.
(1) **Error rate.** 120 printed words (2–5 graphemes long) were individually presented for reading aloud. MC read 2-letter words 100% correctly, 90% with 3- and 4-letter words, and

Table 8–2. The *Schonell Test of Oral Word Reading* (Schonell, 1961)

Test	Pretest*	Posttest**
Accuracy***	79/100	89/100
Time	15:59 min	19:09 min

* given the day prior to the first day of tx

** given on the last day of tx

***Number correct/number possible

Table 8–3. Length test results

		% Accurate	Correct RT*
Pretreatment	Long Words	92.5	7.507
	Short Words	93.3	3.481
Posttreatment	Long Words	64	10.265
	Short Words	90	5.610

*Mean msec

87% with 5-letter words. All errors were in medial (4/10) or final word positions (6/10).

(2) **Response latency.** We developed an additional task for tachistoscopic presentation in which the patient was shown a printed word in his left visual field and requested to read the word aloud. His response time (RT) was measured in the manner described in section III.B.3. Eighty words were presented for unlimited exposure durations, with 40 words that were 3–4 letters long and 40 words that were 7–8 letters long. Pretreatment results can be seen in Table 8–3. MC responded more quickly to short words than to long words.

c. **Spelling regularity.** If MC's reading deficit was not linguistic, but was related to a defect in visual perceptual processing, he should not be influenced by linguistic variables. MC should be able to read irregular words as well as he reads regular words. To test this we used the irregularly spelled word reading subtest from the *Battery of Adult Reading Function* (Rothi, Coslett, & Heilman, 1984). MC was able to read these words (26 correct/

30 possible) as well as regularly spelled words balanced for frequency and length (29 correct/30 possible).

d. **Finally, writing and spelling** as tested on the *Western Aphasia Battery* (Kertesz, 1982) were normal in speed, legibility, and accuracy (see Table 8–1). Although MC's reading was reasonably accurate, it was clearly laborious and effortful and seemed to tax his reportedly limited short-term memory.

In summary, MC displayed alexia characterized by slow, effortful reading of each word of text. When reading words aloud, he spelled aloud and then usually successfully pronounced the word. When asked, he could successfully suppress overt letter naming. No coexisting agraphia was noted.

3. **Implicit Semantic Knowledge Test** (semantic priming in a lexical decision task). This task was designed to assess if MC accessed implicit knowledge about word meaning even when unable to say the word aloud.

   a. **Method**
      (1) **The task** was for the patient to say if a seen stimulus was a word or not. Some of the stimuli were real words and some were nonsense. Before being shown the stimulus, however, the patient was shown another word (called a prime word) that may or may not have been semantically related to the stimulus. The question was: Is the patient faster at identifying words and rejecting nonwords if he has prior knowledge of its potential meaning? For example, can one say the printed word /carrot/ is a "word" faster, if before seeing that word, they were shown the word /vegetable/ (a primed condition) rather than the word /clothes/ (an unprimed condition)?
      (2) **A printed prime** was presented (500 msec) to MC's spared left visual field using a tachistoscope followed by a white screen (500 msec), followed by a word or nonword stimulus that was shown until MC responded verbally with "word" or "not a word."
      (3) **Trials with 80 words and 80 nonwords** for a total of 160 were presented.
      (4) **Using a voice activated relay,** RT was measured from the onset of the stimulus until his verbal response.

   b. **Results.** MC was faster at stating that words were words than at stating that nonwords were nonwords. In the case of stating that words were words, MC demonstrated semantic priming (i.e., RT was faster for semantically primed target words than RT for target words that were not preceded by semantically related words) (see Table 8–4).

IV. DIAGNOSIS

A. The Disorder

This evaluation indicated that MC displayed alexia of the letter-by-letter reading type without agraphia. His aphasia was limited to a visual confrontation naming deficit. Because reading performance was not influenced either by spelling regularity or concreteness, and because of the advantage he displayed for processing real words compared to nonsense on the lexical decision task, we assumed that later lexical stages of word reading were comparatively intact. This was in contrast to the observed early reading stage influences such as MC's sensitivity to word length.

B. Considerations

MC had both a right quadrantanopia and a "recent memory" problem. Although MC displayed a confrontation naming deficit worsened by limiting the visual exposure of the stimuli, relatively little other evidence of aphasia was present.

V. PROGNOSIS

A. Prognostic Signs

1. **Negative prognostic signs:**

    a. **Reports of mild recent memory problems,** possibly indicative of impairment in consolidation of new knowledge, and

    b. **A speech/language pathologist** had treated MC in the previous year and said that MC had reached maximum benefit.

2. **Positive prognostic signs:**

    a. **MC was premorbidly intelligent,**

    b. **No appearance of depression,**

Table 8–4. Semantic priming of a lexical decision task

Word types	Pretest*		Posttest**	
	RT***	Accuracy****	RT***	Accuracy****
Primed Words	1.993	92.5	2.279	87.5
Unprimed Words	2.499	92.5	2.481	87.5
Nonwords	3.527	83.7	2.794	32.5

* Given the day prior to the first day of tx

** Given on the last day of tx

*** Mean msec for response time

****Mean percentage correct

    c. Desired to improve his reading ability,

    d. Suffered a single, lateralized stroke,

    e. No other health problems,

    f. Strong family support, and

    g. MC had never received treatment specifically for his reading problem.

B. Expected Outcome

MC was accepted into our alexia treatment research program, and he was admitted as an inpatient because he lived too far away to commute. This admission was made possible through his participation in a research protocol; under routine circumstances this would not have been authorized.

    1. We predicted MC would not change further without therapy because:

        a. He had likely achieved most of the functional gain expected from physiologic recovery, and

        b. The past clinician had discharged him from further treatment, stating that MC had reached the maximum benefit.

2. **We predicted that the reading treatment** we designed had potential to be effective because:

   a. **This same program** had previously helped a similar patient (Rothi & Moss, 1992),

   b. **MC displayed semantic priming** on a lexical decision task (see section III.B.3.b.), suggesting that he was able to utilize implicit semantic information about words he saw, even when he was prevented from naming letters aloud.

3. **Finally, we felt that after our treatment program,** the patient would be more successful at attempts to read recreationally because we anticipated that he would have faster and greater semantic appreciation of the material as the result of our treatment described in the next section, which would focus on these attributes.

VI. FOCUSING THE TREATMENT

A. Rationale

MC was seen by our service for pretreatment testing, treatment, and posttreatment testing over 2 weeks, with five 30-minute sessions per day (50 total sessions = 25 hours total).

1. **Why treat these patients?** Because individuals with alexia without agraphia may utilize a letter-naming strategy that allows them to read single words, this form of alexia may be seen as less debilitated than alexia with agraphia. Patients with this disorder have relatively little concomitant aphasia and are often able to return to their vocations and live independently. However, we have found that they may remain frustrated by their alexia, because their letter naming strategy is slow and prone to error when letters are misidentified, with successful reading limited by the length of the material being read, and some patients unable to read more than single words or single, short sentences in text.

2. **What kind of treatment?** Landis, Regard, and Serrat (1980) reported a person with reading problems similar to MC who, immediately after his stroke, could classify words semantically that he was unable to read aloud. This patient subsequently developed a letter-naming strategy that allowed him to name words aloud. However, as this strategy emerged, the patient lost the initial ability to

classify words based on meaning. Letter naming may be a strategy that permits deficient readers to compensate for an inability to arrive at a whole-word form percept explicitly (Speedie et al., 1982). However, this compensation may interfere with the capability of attaining at least some level of word understanding directly. Therefore the focus of therapy reported in this chapter was to reduce such interference by preventing letter naming and encouraging the emergence of direct access to word meaning. This treatment was successful in improving reading (defined as access to meaning) in our previously studied case (Rothi & Moss, 1992); the therapy for MC attempted to replicate it. Goals of the treatment were to:

a. **Prevent MC from identifying each letter** of a word visually. This was accomplished by rapid tachistoscopic, word presentation to MC's normal visual field. Rapid presentation was assumed to prevent MC from using a letter-by-letter reading strategy and to force him to inspect the whole word form.

b. **Direct MC to semantically process words.**

B. Methods and Results

Two treatment tasks were used. In both, MC was told he would be shown a printed word and "Don't tell me the names of the words you will see, just tell me what category they belong to." When he achieved 80% accuracy at one presentation rate, exposure duration was dropped by 100 msec increments.

1. Word Category Discrimination Treatment

a. Method
(1) **The corpus** used during each therapy session included 40 words randomly selected each session from a larger corpus of 100 stimuli within the five semantic categories.
(2) **Thirty total sessions** of exposure of these 40 printed words via tachistoscope to the left visual field for limited durations;
(3) **After stimulus presentation,** MC was asked if the word belonged to one of two categories "X" or "Y" (i.e., "vegetable" or "clothes") included in the central corpus. That is, if he saw "carrot" he was asked: "Is this a vegetable or clothes?" The clinician recorded MC's accuracy and the reaction time, RT (as described in section III.B.3.).

(4) **After each trial** MC was immediately told by the clinician whether he was correct/incorrect; when incorrect, he was told the correct category.

b. Results

(1) **We began this task initially establishing exposure durations.** We decided to accept an exposure 100 msec longer than the shortest exposure, yielding at least 70% accuracy, which was 900 msec.

(2) **Our intent was to lower the exposure duration** during the course of therapy and we were able to do so. MC progressed nicely, with final presentation rates approaching 600 msec.

(3) **At 600 msec,** we were confident that MC was not able to utilize a letter naming strategy, because this duration is too short to allow identification of each letter. Whereas, we had evidence from MC's performance on the Implicit Semantic Knowledge Test (section III.B.3.) that he was capable of accessing the meaning of words he could not name, his performance accuracy never stabilized at this speed and he never was able to identify word category for these rapidly presented printed words.

2. Word Category Naming Treatment

a. Method

(1) **Printed words** were shown via tachistoscope to the left visual field for limited durations (described below) and MC was asked to say aloud the semantic category for each. For example, he saw the printed word /carrot/ and was to say aloud the superordinate category the stimulus belonged to (i.e., "vegetable"). Both response accuracy and RT were recorded.

(2) **In each session** (24 total sessions) 40 stimuli were presented randomly selected from the corpus of 100 stimuli described previously.

(3) **We began initially with three training sessions** in which exposure duration was long enough to accommodate MC's letter naming reading strategy (5 seconds). He was told "correct" or "incorrect" by the clinician immediately after his response. For incorrect responses, he was informed of the correct category.

b. Results

(1) **Therapy sessions began with exposure durations** of 900 msec at which speed MC was able to correctly name the stimulus category at least 50% of the time.

(2) **In contrast to the Word Category Discrimination Treatment,** MC never progressed with decremental changes in exposure duration on this task because his accuracy remained variable and never reached criterion. However, 20% accuracy would be chance performance on this task and his performance remained above that at 900 msec. In addition, 900 msec exposure duration would clearly impede a letter-by-letter reading strategy. One could conclude that while MC did not become better able to explicitly access the meaning of seen words, he did retain his pre-existing level of implicit semantic access.

C. Outcome Measures

The following tasks were measured the day before treatment began and following MC's final treatment session.

1. **Implicit Semantic Knowledge Test.** (For methods, see section III.B.3.) Response time was measured, with the prediction that, if therapy worked, this patient would demonstrate increasing sensitivity to the semantic prime, either by responding more accurately or with shorter RTs. The lexical decision for the nonprimed words and nonwords would have equivalent RTs because there was no advantage for a primed meaning. From the data, it would appear that although MC responded to semantic primes for seen words before therapy, semantic priming was no longer evident after therapy.

2. *Boston Naming Test-Modified.* (For methods, see section III.B.1.d.) We hypothesized that MC's reading and confrontation naming deficits emanated from a common perceptual problem. Therefore we predicted that our reading therapy would improve picture naming as well. Response time and accuracy were recorded, as was the actual response so that errors could be later coded as semantic approximations or "other" error type. Before treatment, MC scored 7 correct/60 possible on this task. Ten of 53 error responses were in some way semantically related to the target. MC's posttreatment performance was relatively unchanged; he scored 4 correct/60 possible with 7 error responses providing some target-relevant, semantic information. This contrasts with pretreatment

scores on the unmodified form of the *Boston Naming Test* (see section III.B.1.c.), on which MC gave related semantic information in 80% of errors.

3. **Word Length Test.** (For methods see section III.B.2.b.). We predicted that if therapy was effective in disengaging MC from his letter-by-letter reading strategy, he would no longer be influenced by word length. In fact, the data suggest that MC became less accurate and took longer to read aloud longer words (when compared to shorter words) subsequent to treatment.

VII. DISCUSSION

MC did not respond to the Category Naming Treatment Test, but did respond to the Category Discrimination Treatment Test. On the latter, he continued to meet criterion performance and we were able to progressively lower the stimulus exposure durations. In general, however, the treatment programs were not effective in improving MC's reading of untreated materials. Almost all measures of word reading (word length, semantic priming, category decision) showed a worsening of performance after treatment.

A. Rationale

1. **Regarding the theoretical rationale** of this particular treatment approach, it has been noted that patients can provide information (e.g., priming effects) about objects or faces they claim not to recognize in agnosia (Bauer, 1993) as well as in cases of acquired amnesia (Schacter, 1987) and other syndromes such as blindsight (Weiskrantz, 1986). What relationship does this implicit form of semantic information have to the explicit system? Are they completely unrelated (modular) systems in which implicit knowledge cannot be recruited to support a dysfunctional explicit system? The answer to this question remains in dispute (see Sherry & Schacter, 1987, for one version), but the success of our approach with our previously reported case (Rothi & Moss, 1992) would speak against the pessimistic proposition that the implicit knowledge cannot be recruited to support explicit semantic access.

2. **Why would we continue to pursue a treatment that did not appear to be progressing for 30 sessions?** Remember that a similar patient had used this approach successfully, and MC's intervention was part of a larger research initiative. Because there was a

possibility that MC simply required longer exposure to the techniques, we continued on through the (a priori) specified length of the research protocol (2 weeks) and tried to manipulate exposure durations in the hopes of sparking a positive response.

B. Alternatives

What are the differences between MC and the case successfully treated (Rothi & Moss, 1992)?

1. **The Rothi and Moss (1992) case** was seen twice per day (45–60 minute sessions) for two weeks, with MC seen 5 times per day (30-minute sessions) for 2 weeks. One possibility is that MC's treatment schedule may have been too intensive and that fatigue might have negatively influenced the results.

2. **During the 50 sessions** MC never learned the route to our laboratory; our previous case independently drove 40 miles each day to treatment sessions. Might MC's "topographic amnesia" reflect a form of memory disorder that precludes the use of some visually based abilities that were available in our previous case?

3. **Reports of recent memory problems** by MC's wife and his inability to remember more than the current president and 0/3 objects for 3 minutes may reflect a significant memory disorder that we did not test for. The Rothi and Moss (1992) patient did not have a problem with memory. How MC's memory deficit might have contributed to his treatment failure is unclear. However, in retrospect we should have considered the role of memory in this training procedure (see Helm-Estabrooks, this volume).

4. **Is it possible that MC was more severely alexic** than the Rothi and Moss (1992) case? We cannot compare these cases on accuracy or efficiency of the letter-by-letter strategy, as we did not assess the influence of word length on reading time in the Rothi and Moss (1992) case. We do know, however, that it took the Rothi and Moss (1992) case 2 minutes to read 10 words (5 letters or less), suggesting that he was possibly even slower at reading words aloud than MC. Although not a direct comparison of alexia severity across the two, this does imply that MC was not worse than the Rothi and Moss (1992) case and that alexia severity cannot explain his lack of response to the treatment.

Might he then have been *too mild* to show an effective response to the treatment? MC did show a significant degree of alexia in that, in the context of reading major lexical items 5 letters in length printed in bold type presented one at a time for unlimited durations, his error rate was 13%. As all of these words were below the 8th grade reading level, this seems to be a very high level of error for a college graduate. In addition, one would wonder why the patient, if he did not respond to the treatment, was made worse by the intervention? Wouldn't we predict that the semantic analysis of words would still emerge when he was prevented from using his letter-by-letter strategy? Therefore, there is only a limited possibility that the degree of alexia that MC displayed was so mild that it inhibited his ability to respond to the treatment.

5. **MC displayed a right superior quadrantanopia,** with the Rothi and Moss (1992) case displaying a right inferior quadrantanopia. Upper quadrant deficits are associated with ventral temporal occipital lesions and lower quadrant deficits are associated with dorsal occipital parietal lesions. The ventral and dorsal systems may mediate different visual gnostic functions (Ungerleider & Mishkin, 1982). That is, Ungerleider and Mishkin (1982) proposed that two pathways feed forward from the occipital lobe: a dorsal system important for recognizing "where" stimuli are in space and a ventral system that assists in recognizing "what" seen stimuli are. The Rothi and Moss (1992) case had a quadrant defect associated with dorsal lesions implying that the "what" system was intact and the "where" system was damaged. In contrast, MC had a defect that would imply that the "where" system was intact and the "what" system was damaged. Might this difference in lesion loci be the difference in responsiveness to this treatment approach? Might one need the "what" system to utilize implicit semantic information?

6. **MC displayed a visual confrontation naming deficit** that was seen when picture stimuli were presented rapidly. Although the Rothi and Moss (1992) case was not aphasic, we did not test his picture naming ability using rapid presentations and do not know if he had a similar problem (see Hillis & Caramazza, 1995, for a thorough discussion of vision-specific naming disorders).

7. **Finally, we looked at the nature of the errors** MC produced on the *Boston Naming Test* (Kaplan et al., 1983). When exposure durations were manipulated, MC appeared to have access to far more semantic information with long exposure times than he did when

the durations were limited to 500 msec. If we found that visual confrontation naming ability and word reading ability were compromised from a common genesis (see section VII.B.6.), and if MC developed semantic information about pictures only after 500 msec as seen on the BNT performance, our treatment may not only have prevented a letter-by-letter reading strategy, but eliminated specification of the semantic representation also. Why MC's access to semantic information would be so abnormally delayed or require a longer visual exposure of the stimulus than normally required is unclear.

C. Hindsight

1. **Outcome.** One wonders if this intervention actually hurt MC's remaining reading ability. However, because MC spontaneously reverted to a letter-by-letter reading strategy when given unlimited exposure durations, we believed that he would reinstitute this compensatory strategy with time. During follow-up phone conversations (every 6 months for 2 years) MC and his wife were asked about his reading and they reported no lasting harm from the treatment.

2. **Cost.** How realistic would it be that one could implement treatments like these within the typical clinical milieu (e.g., the lack of a tachistoscope or computer)? We do not recommend treatments like these be done as inpatients, or as intensively as done in this case. We (Rothi & Moss, 1992) have provided this treatment successfully to an outpatient, and although we continue to believe that daily treatments are needed, we do not recommend exceeding 60 minutes per day. In addition, we have found that a treatment program based upon these principles (limit exposure duration and emphasize semantic processing of the printed stimuli) can be easily implemented using words printed on 3" × 5" cards (i.e., "flash cards") shown for 1 second at a time (as per clinician estimate). Response times can be scored by a stopwatch. This type of program could easily be modified for home use and performed at home by caregivers or friends—therefore drastically reducing the cost of such a program.

3. **How might we do things differently now?**

   a. **Is it possible to manipulate the exposure duration** of the target stimulus to minimize the opportunity for MC to segment the word visually while simultaneously allowing enough time so that he can develop a semantic representation? We might try to show the target word for short durations repeatedly. The short exposures (500 mscc) might prevent the patient from visually segmenting the word but the recurrent exposure might allow a semantic representation to build. Using the tachistoscope, for example, one could show the target for 500 msec, followed by a white screen for 500 msec, followed by a repetition of this cycle until the patient felt he could respond with the category name with some level of confidence. Using 3" × 5" cards, the target could simply be exposed for a second, covered, and re-exposed repeatedly in the same manner. Of course, this method remains untested as it is not clear that repeated short exposures will allow a person to develop a semantic representation for seen items.

b. **If, in fact, further research shows that this treatment** is not effective in individuals who have deficient "what" recognition, we would then recommend that those with superior quadrant visual field cuts, such as MC, be treated with other methods, such as the approach described by Beeson in Chapter 7.

4. We believe the major lesson learned from MC is that **not all cases of alexia without agraphia or more specifically not all cases of letter-by-letter reading disorders are the same nor should they be treated in the same manner.** MC did display implicit access to semantic information as a letter-by-letter reader. Our previous experience suggested that he should have responded to the treatment we designed; that is, if we used his ability to implicitly access semantic information as an indicator of his candidacy for the treatment. Obviously, we have learned that this visual perceptual portion of the reading system does not function quite that simply. Why MC showed access to implicit semantic knowledge (as in the case of the semantic priming of the lexical decision task), but performed on the *Boston Naming Test–Modified* as though explicit semantic knowledge was deficient for visual material seen for less than 500 msec, is not clear. The relationship between implicit and explicit forms of semantic knowledge remains a mystery. The more we can learn about it from a functional/anatomic perspective, the more precise we may become in designing and choosing efficacious approaches to treatment and functional compensation. This remains our challenge for the future: to further explicate the visual perceptual portion of the reading system in all its complexity (including how one accesses implicit as well as explicit levels of semantic knowledge);

to attempt this and alternative treatments such as the one described by Beeson in Chapter 7 in a variety of cases whose visual systems are well studied; and ultimately to consider which functional and/ or anatomic attributes of a case predict which treatments will be more efficacious before they are instituted.

VIII. ACKNOWLEDGMENT

We wish to acknowledge the support of this research project by the Neurology Service, Gainesville VAMC and Rehabilitation Research and Development Service, Department of Veterans Affairs. In addition, we wish to thank Kenneth M. Heilman, M.D., for his help in the conceptual development of this treatment program as well as his helpful comments regarding this manuscript.

IX. REFERENCES

Bauer, R. (1993). Agnosia. In K. M. Heilman & E. Valenstein (Eds.), *Clinical neuropsychology* (pp. 215–277). New York: Oxford University Press.

Bub, D., Black, S., & Behrmann, M. (1987). New evidence for unconscious reading in pure alexia. Academy of Aphasia, Phoenix.

Coslett, H. B., & Saffran, E. M. (1994). Mechanisms of implicit reading in alexia. In M. J. Farah & G. Ratcliff (Eds.), *The neuropsychology of high-level vision: Collected tutorial essays* (pp. 299–330). Hillsdale, NJ: Lawrence Erlbaum.

Déjerine, K. (1891). Sur un cas de cecite verbal avec agraphie suivi d'autopsie. *Memories de la Société de Biologie, 3,* 197–201.

Déjerine, K. (1892). Contribution a l'etude anatomochimique des differentes varietes de cecite verbale. *Compte Rendu Hebdomadaire des Sceances et Memoires de la Société de Biologie, 4,* 61–90.

Ellis, A. W., Young, A. W., & Anderson, C. (1988). Modes of word recognition in the left and right cerebral hemispheres. *Brain and Language, 35,* 254–273.

Henderson, L. (1987). Word recognition: A tutorial review. In M. Coltheart (Ed.), *Attention and performance. XII: The psychology of reading* (pp. 171–200). Hillsdale: NJ: Lawrence Erlbaum.

Hillis, A. E., & Caramazza, A. (1995). Cognitive and neural mechanisms underlying visual and semantic processing: Implications from "optic aphasia." *Journal of Cognitive Neuroscience, 7,* 457–478.

Kaplan, E., Goodglass, H., & Weintraub, S. (1983). *Boston Naming Test.* Philadelphia: Lea & Febiger.

Kertesz, A. (1982). *Western Aphasia Battery.* San Antonio, TX: The Psychological Corporation.

Landis, T., Regard, M., & Serrat, A. (1980). Iconic reading in a case of alexia without agraphia caused by a brain tumor: A tachistoscopic study. *Brain and Language, 11,* 45–53.

Paivio, A., Yuille, J. C., & Madigan, S. A. (1968). Concreteness, imagery and mean-ingfulness values for 925 nouns. *Journal of Experimental Psychology, 76* (Suppl.), 1–25.

Rothi, L. J. G., Coslett, H. B., & Heilman, K. M. (1984). *Battery of adult reading function* (exp. ed.). Unpublished.

Rothi, L. J. G., & Moss, S. (1992). Alexia without agraphia: Potential for model assisted therapy. *Clinics in Communication Disorders, 2,* 11–18.

Schacter, D. L. (1987). Implicit memory: History and current status. *Journal of Experimental Psychology (Learning, Memory and Cognition), 13,* 501–518.

Schonell, F. J. (1961). *The psychology and teaching of reading* (pp. 258–263). New York: Philosophical Library.

Shallice, T., & Saffran, E. (1986). Lexical processing in the absence of explicit word identification: Evidence from a letter-by-letter reader. *Cognitive Neuropsychology, 3,* 429–458.

Sherry, D. F., & Schacter, D. L. (1987). The evolution of multiple memory systems. *Psychological Review, 94,* 439–454.

Speedie, L., Rothi, L. J., & Heilman, K. M. (1982). Spelling dyslexia: A form of cross-cuing. *Brain and Language, 15,* 340–352.

Spreen, O., & Strauss, E. (1991). *A compendium of neuropsychological tests.* New York: Oxford University Press.

Thorndike, E. L., & Lorge, I. (1968). *The teacher's word book of 30,000 words.* New York: Bureau of Publications, Columbia University.

Ungerleider, L. G., & Mishkin, M. (1982). Two cortical visual systems. In D. J. Ingle, M. A. Goodale, & R. J. W. Mansfield (Eds.), *Analysis of visual behavior* (pp. 549–586). Cambridge, MA: MIT Press.

Weiskrantz, L. (1986). *Blindsight: A case study and implications.* New York: Oxford University Press.

CHAPTER

9

Treating Real-Life Functionality in a Couple Coping With Severe Aphasia

JON G. LYON, Ph.D.

I. BACKGROUND

A. Introduction

1. The Nature of this Treatment Case

This treatment case stands apart in several distinct ways from those that use traditional methods of managing aphasia. First, it targets change in the communication of a married couple challenged by the wife's severe aphasia, rather than focusing on her language and communication alone. Second, it targets their communication at home, rather than in a clinic. Third, it focuses on helping these people feel personally connected rather than just facilitating an exchange of information. Thus, this treatment is foremost one of persons interacting with one another rather than a prescriptive list of tasks aimed at overcoming language dysfunction. This treatment's aim is to restore harmony to daily life, not simply to repair "broken parts" within an injured party's communication system.

The prime constructs of this treatment are different from those of traditional therapy as well. Instead of the treatment targets being adequacy, efficiency, or proficiency in the exchange of information, they are, instead, establishing comfort, ease, confidence, and pleasure interacting with one another. This therapeutic bias toward bonding interactants, though, does not mean that exchanging information is not involved or important. It simply means that improving the exchange of content is only valuable when it is overlaid on a known and operative means of keeping its interactants mutually bonded. Individuals confronting severe aphasia first must feel connected as people who care for one another, before they can begin to incorporate more proficient ways of repairing or circumventing linguistic or communicative breakdowns. According to this model of treatment, being communicatively accurate or understood is important only to the extent that it unifies interactants as sharers of experience, feeling, or thought. When therapy inadvertently isolates people in the exchanging of information rather than bringing them closer together, its real-life value diminishes.

The purpose of this case presentation is not to offer a precise or proven treatment methodology. In fact, we need to spend more time exploring treatment methods in natural settings to learn what may or may not enhance communicative effectiveness at home before vesting heavily in their measurement (Lyon, 1996). This case description demonstrates how I attempted to enhance the personal connectedness and exchange of information in a couple whose daily existence was shaken to its most basic levels of function and survival by severe aphasia.

2. Treatment Beginning

I met this couple long after standard reimbursable care had ended. What is even more important, however, is that the type of therapy described here would not been a part of standard care even if the need had been identified earlier. The absence of such remediation is not out of neglect or lack of awareness, but due to a difference in philosophy, perspective, and history of aphasia's treatment. Although clinicians have long sought methods to improve functional communication and well-being in the daily lives of people confronting the complications of severe aphasia, the roots of this care and the delivery system in America lie in a medical model. In this model, repair of the underlying language impairment represented the best and most expeditious means of improving associated communicative functions in real life. This approach assumes that by remediating the source of the problem *in* a patient and *in* the clinic, any gains that accrue will carry over to real life, thereby improving its quality.

More recently, though, managed care administrators have begun asking for proof that clinically based treatments do, indeed, have an impact on real-life functions and quality of life. Unfortunately, there is little hard evidence with which to argue such a case, and, as a result, it remains unclear if our past treatment practices will endure. It is not that traditional therapies have failed to show any real-life relevancies—they have! It is that clinically based treatments have failed to make communication in everyday life a priority from their initiation. At best, functionality in natural settings has been a concluding afterthought to clinical repair of an underlying language or communication disorder. Now we are faced with a different set of health care rules for reimbursement. With these, there is increased urgency to develop and use therapies that blend clinical and real-life objectives from their outset.

3. Treatment Course and Duration

Even after deciding to institute such real-life oriented therapies, the challenge remains in prescribing their optimal course and duration. Enhancing personal connectedness in a couple coping with severe aphasia is likely a protracted task, a prospect not favored under managed care. However, there is no single or "correct" prescriptive answer for merging current funding constraints into a treatment formula that assures functionality of communication in real life. As illustrated in this case, therapy entailed a series of clinical and home adaptations extending over several months and requiring weekly sessions and modifications.

Such treatment cost, even if documented and shown to influence functional communication and quality of life, would not likely qualify for reimbursement under current health care guidelines (see

Frattali's Chapter 10). Treatment began long postonset and its objectives emphasized parameters of communication not confined only to the injured adult but to them as husband and wife. However, if speech-language pathologists are to remain a part of the treatment process, we need to shift and look beyond clinical repair from the beginning of therapy, and allot time and support to managing the social dilemmas of people coping with aphasia in real life. To do this, we must turn to treatments outside clinical domains, not simply because managed care is forcing us in this direction, but because these methods are the most direct and the most potent force for eliciting the changes we seek. Finally, we need to act immediately and decisively to ensure that we remain participants in a therapeutic process that may otherwise cease.

B. Conceptual Framework

1. The Scope of Aphasia Treatment

Change in the health care system is not the only influence pushing aphasia treatment in new or different directions. There has been a growing awareness among clinical researchers that we must attend to more than the linguistic impairment of aphasia (Frattali, 1996; Holland, 1992; Kagan, 1995b). The additional factors in this treatment formula are what the World Health Organization (WHO, 1980) has termed the "disability" and the "handicap" of chronic dysfunction.

"Disability" is the functional consequence that follows in daily life from aphasia's underlying language impairment. The use of communication in daily life has become the reimbursable criterion of today's health care system. Providers are assessing the net worth of therapies by their ability to enact immediate, verifiable, and lasting changes in everyday life (Frattali, 1996; Warren, 1996). As a result, treatments and assessment measures have begun to focus on the management of disabilities, or "functional aspects" of aphasia (Elman & Bernstein-Ellis, 1995; Frattali, 1996). However, within this attempt to target the resumption of function in daily life, however, little attention has been given to the extent of a patient's handicap (Lyon, 1992; Simmons-Mackie & Damico, in press).

"Handicap" is the personal and social consequence of aphasia's disability. When characterized this way, it may seem that a handicap is a therapeutic step removed from the seemingly more important, functional applications of daily life. It may appear that restoring communication at home requires eliminating its disabling features first, not so much coping with its social consequences. However, overcoming the disability is not a process separate or removed from bringing people closer together through words. Communication serves dual purposes: to unite people and to exchange information. When talking is no longer possible as a means of exchange, as with people confronting severe aphasia, the inability to remain personally bonded may be more devastating than the inability to exchange content. Under such circumstances, interactants may need to be shown ways of merging as individuals who care for one another (overcoming the handicap), as much as methods for perfecting the exchange of content (overcoming the disability).

Restoring a personal bridge between people with aphasia and their loved ones is not a process that is separate from exchanging information. Both aspects, personal connecting and information sharing, must exist to some degree for communication to take place and remain ongoing. However to date, aphasia treatments have predominately targeted the exchange of content while ignoring the social connecting of interactants. To understand the prescription of the treatment that follows, it is crucial to understand how exchanging content and the social connecting of participants interact to create functional communication in real-life settings.

2. Relating Disability and Handicap to Functional Communication

Simmons-Mackie (Simmons, 1993) used direct observation and the videotaping of interactions to study the communicative exchanges of two adults with moderate/severe aphasia interacting with typical interactants in their natural settings. Both subjects were more than 1 year postonset and had undergone traditional speech-language therapy; one was still receiving out-patient therapy. In terms of participant observation, 14½ hours of interaction were analyzed in 17 different contexts. The videotaping analyses involved 8½ hours across 22 different contexts. Interviewing interactants and cross-observations of taped segments by other trained observers were also a significant aspect of the data collection.

Simmons-Mackie's findings are noteworthy in many ways, but particularly her observations of communicative use. Her subjects displayed a preference for strategies in conversation that bonded them personally with others, a function she referred to as "interactional," rather than "transactional," or an attempt to convey the content of the message. That is, the two subjects with aphasia frequently entered conversations to bond with others rather than **just** to impart information. If functionality in natural settings is our ultimate treatment target, then we need to equally address the use of communication for purposes of social interaction.

3. Accounting for Transactional and Interactional Aspects of Communication in Treatment

It has been noted that normal conversation is comprised of both "interacting" and "transacting" forms of communication (Kagan, 1995b). Sometimes we feel as if exchanging information (transacting) is the more prominent part of daily conversations. However, if we reflect on what really impacts our lives, a lot of the informational content in our messages can be sacrificed over time with minimal effect on our main message or our well-being. For example, we do need to know the airline and time of arrival if we are about to pick up a friend at the airport, but sharing small talk about the flight, such as the air turbulence over the Rockies, the stale peanuts, or the conversation with a talkative traveler, are typically social niceties that hold us together during the ride home. Few of us would describe social bonding with another person as conversationally unimportant, but knowing the particulars of a friend's arrival is absolutely essential. Once properly noted, though, it allows conversants to return to topics that bind rather than contain important details. It is this interactional connection that lasts long after each person has returned home and we've forgotten about the transactional details that were once important.

In severe aphasia, both interactional and transactional forms of communication abruptly cease in any apparent form. Without access to a mutually understood "transactional code," conversants struggle to find a common, reliable way to connect and share. This struggle typically produces great discomfort in both the person who is aphasic and the interactant with typical, undamaged communication ability. Besides failing to understand why speech is absent, there is no immediate substitute to take its place. Within this framework, it is not surprising that speech-language pathologists have sought to repair functional language and communication: to find, develop, and implement alternative methods for transacting information.

"Total communication" is a clinically based technique for augmenting spoken transactional aspects of communication in people with severe aphasia. This therapy depends on the implementation of a patient-specific blend of gestural, written, drawn, and visual linguistic/nonlinguistic aids. Much of this therapy is targeted at a patient and carried out within a clinical setting. Its prime purpose is to provide a transactional base from which interactants might share a joint "topic," or "referent." That is, by learning a combined use of speech, gesture, print, and drawing, the person with aphasia is able to share a level of content otherwise not possible through speech alone.

In the treatment case described here, the importance of exploring "total communication" is not questioned. What is in question, though, is whether targeting these techniques to the exclusion of first establishing a personal bondedness between interactants, may unintentionally block access to optimal functionality. Simmons-Mackie (Simmons, 1993) found little evidence of the use of clinically trained communication strategies in the daily conversations of her two subjects with aphasia. What were present, though, were self-styled renditions of these strategies that appeared to meet the personalized needs of the individuals involved. The least used strategies were those that communicatively isolated one interactant from the other instead of linking them as mutual and equal participants in a dynamic, ongoing give-and-take process—strategies such as communication solely through picture boards or word lists.

Thus, it may be that the lack of generalization of clinically based total communication treatments to natural setting is not because of inadequate training of nonspeech modality use. It may be, instead, that transactional treatment targets, although important to the general integrity of communication, must fit within a framework of social bondedness to take hold and flourish. For this reason, it may be far more important to first uncover ways of merging interactants as people sharing a process and then to build on their skills for exchanging content. If this is true, then our insistence on augmentative methods that aid in a contextual exchange of information while separating interactants as people who care for one another may only detract from, rather than remediate, the very process we hope to resolve.

4. An Alternative Framework for Enhancing Communication in Natural Settings

Although communication requires a mutually agreed on code with which to share information, it only requires rudimentary skills to bond interactants personally and socially. It is this function—the bringing together of interactants as individuals sharing with one another before perfection of the use of the code—that characterizes the treatment here. The integrity of merging interactants as communicators in a shared communicative process is not based on how completely, accurately, efficiently, or proficiently information is exchanged. It depends, instead, on how both parties perceive themselves within that exchange and whether they feel equal, comfortable, able, and participatory. This mutuality of participation does not translate into equality of communicative burden, responsibility, or form. In fact, the interactant who is not aphasic typically must assume a far greater percentage of the communicative responsibility to allow the person with severe aphasia to gain equal participatory footing. Equal participation in this therapeutic framework means that for every communicative act by the nonaphasic interactant, a valued response is given by the person with aphasia. As such, the measure of therapeutic worth in this treatment is ease, freedom, and degree of communicative turn-taking, not simply the completeness or accuracy of content.

Therapy begins with establishing a means whereby interactants can comfortably alternate communicative turns. When this shared process becomes successful, treatment shifts toward enhancing participants' skills in exchanging content. However, any development of a broader "transactional" repertoire must complement and fit within the then-existing interactional style. If the use of "total communication" techniques threaten a couple's ability to sustain an interactive equality, then the use of these techniques for transactional purposes must be modified. In this way, transactional aspects constantly remain in the background, with interactional aspects remaining in the foreground of the communicative process. That is not to say that an exchange of information is absent or unimportant, but that it is secondary to the goal of keeping participants actively bonded in a communicative process that is mutually satisfying.

One way to put this therapy into perspective is to compare it with prior treatment in this case. Even though it was extensive, previous remediation was devoted to the repair and circumvention of the wife's language and communication dysfunctions. When supported by a clinician in a clinical setting, this woman had become a somewhat consistent user of a picture board to express basic needs and wants. Yet this aid failed to enhance communication at home either as a means of exchanging content or as a means of merging the wife and husband as conversational partners. In contrast, the treatment described here established a communicative turn-taking process first by initially de-emphasizing the extent and adequacy of information exchanged and by instead fostering interactive successes in a mutual give-and-take process. The specifics of that treatment process follows.

II. THE TREATED COUPLE

A. Our Introduction to One Another

This treatment couple is a 64-year-old woman with severe aphasia and her 63-year-old husband, referred to here as Betty and Hal. I met Betty and Hal at a group session I was overseeing at the May 1996 meeting of "Opening Doors," an international gathering of adults with aphasia and their caregivers held annually in Ann Arbor, MI. The topic of the session was active participation in daily life, during which participants were asked to rate their own personal involvement on a 10-point scale.

As I attempted to facilitate their responses, it was apparent that this task was not comprehensible to Betty. She repetitively recited one of her few stereotypical phrases, "I don't know." Despite my efforts to orient her to the task by introducing visual aids, simplifying my language, gesturing, printing words, and drawing, nothing worked. She was attentive, but obviously not benefiting from my attempt at total communication, so I decided to move on and to meet with the couple afterwards. At that meeting, I learned that they resided 90 miles from my clinic in south-central Wisconsin and we arranged to meet there in early July.

B. Biography

Betty and Hal met in 1954 and were married the following year. Betty had been married previously and was caring for two young daughters. Both Betty and Hal were high school graduates. Hal was a state highway patrolman. Over the next 3 years, they added two more daughters to the family. Betty worked at home and raised the four children, with Hal employed in law enforcement and criminal investigation.

When the children reached high school age, Betty took a half-time position as a sales clerk. She remained in that position for the next 16 years. Retiring in 1986, she filled her week by babysitting two preschool grandchildren in her home. Although the grandchildren had begun school by the time she suffered her stroke in March of 1995, she continued to care for them before and after school hours.

Hal continued his law enforcement career as an investigative officer for the State of Wisconsin Justice Department and retired in 1988 after

30 years. Following retirement, he was frequently away from the house during the day, attending to his aged mother and engaged in other activities and interests, such as playing golf.

C. Medical History

Betty had a history of treated hypertension and suffered an occlusive left middle cerebral artery infarction on March 16, 1995. In addition to her aphasia, she was left with dense right hemiplegia. At 1 month postonset, a CT scan of the brain was read as showing a large temporal, parietal, and posterior frontal lobe infarction extending subcortically into the internal capsule and basal ganglia. There were signs of small, isolated pockets of acute hemorrhaging that appeared to be subsequent to the initial occlusive insult, but a CT scan at the time of the injury had failed to show any signs of hemorrhage. There were no neuroradiographic or clinical findings to suggest that Betty's infarction extended beyond the left cerebral hemisphere.

D. Prior Treatment

Betty was seen by a speech-language pathologist toward the end the first week of hospitalization. She was initially unresponsive when admitted, "awakening" only days prior to being transferred to a regional rehabilitation center. From March 24 through May 19, 1995, she received speech-language, physical, and occupational therapies twice daily at the center. She was described initially as "globally aphasic," that is, with severe dysfunction across all language modalities. Treatment involved traditional receptive/expressive language stimulation drill. Throughout the first 2 months of therapy, Betty made slow but steady improvements. Her identification of pictured objects in a field of two progressed from no response to 80% accuracy. A combination of cues (auditory with printed words and auditory with gestures) were the most facilitative in aiding Betty's comprehension. She began imitating short, high-frequency words but spontaneous speech remained nonfunctional with a few intelligible stereotypes and inconsistent and unreliable use of "Okay" and "No."

She continued therapy as an outpatient at the same rehabilitation center from May 19 through June 23, 1995. Hour-long treatment sessions were initially provided three times weekly, but soon reduced to two, and then one, because of "an absence of change" in her performance. Hal reported that at no time in this 4 month regimen of speech-language services did formal therapy target their communication as a couple. In September 1995, Betty began therapy at a speech-language clinic at a nearby university and completed two semesters of individual therapy and group therapy before coming to my clinic. Individual therapy at the university clinic emphasized a multimodality language stimulation approach, along with continuing work on auditory comprehension and verbal expression, reading and writing tasks. Group therapy appeared to be a combination of language and peer interaction activities. Again, Hal reported no formal treatment as a couple.

III. APPRAISAL

A. Rationale

When Betty and Hal arrived in my clinic early in July, it was apparent that their greatest anguish lay in their inability to communicatively interact with one another in any meaningful and sustainable form. Although Betty's language and communicative skills had improved, she and Hal remained distant and noninteractive as a couple. Each expressed in separate ways their frustration and sorrow in the lack of personal and social closeness. Most difficult was their utter inability to repair communication breakdowns.

The first problem I faced in assessment was quantifying their communicative impairment before treatment so that I could measure change after therapy. Existing standardized measures appeared either too insensitive or nonspecific to capture the type of change anticipated from the type of therapy we were undertaking. Even nonstandardized measures targeted at these interactive realms of communication were nonexistent. So to clarify the issue of measurement, it was important to review the treatment objectives proposed.

1. Short-Term Objectives (first 3 months)

a. **Establishing a means of communicative interaction** that would permit Betty and Hal to feel more personally connected and comfortable in each other's presence.

b. **Developing strategies** that would lessen their communicative anguish and aid in an amicable resolution of life's daily problems.

c. **Increasing the pleasure** that Betty and Hal derived from communication and decreasing feelings of avoidance, duty, burden, or hopelessness.

2. Long-Term Objectives (3 to 12 months)

a. Helping to increase Betty and Hal's participation in daily life.

b. Helping this couple establish more self-determined lifestyles.

Betty was restricted in her participation and independence in daily life because of her severe aphasia and hemiplegia, but Hal was equally restricted! His dysfunction was not because he couldn't act in his own behalf, but because of his perceived obligation to attend to every nuance of Betty's needs and wishes.

B. Measures

Given these treatment objectives, two types of measurement were chosen. In an attempt to capture treatment effects or related changes from treatment, selections were made from standardized assessment tools. For language change, I used *The Boston Assessment of Severe Aphasia* (BASA); for communication change, the ASHA *Functional Assessment of Communicative Skills* (FACS) was selected; for psychosocial well-being, I used the *Affect Balance Scale* (ABS). But, because these measures did not address the interactive anguish of this couple's communication, two additional, nonstandardized measures were added: the *Interactive Communication Scales* (ICS), and the *Psychosocial Well-Being Index* (PWI). These measures are summarized.

1. Standardized Measures

a. Language: *The Boston Assessment of Severe Aphasia* (Helm-Estabrooks, Ramsberger, Morgan, & Nicholas, 1989). This measure has proven highly sensitive in the documentation of basic linguistic and communicative skills in patients exhibiting severe aphasia. Frequently, as these authors note, standard comprehensive tests of aphasia fail to sample the lower continuum of linguistic and nonlinguistic functions. To provide a more inclusive and reliable range in which to judge the ability of adults with severe aphasia, these authors offer a standardized sampling of functions across a variety of realms: auditory comprehension, praxis, oral-gestural expression, reading comprehension, and "other items," which include drawing.

b. Communication: *ASHA Functional Assessment of Communicative Skills* (Frattali, Thompson, Holland, Wohl, &

Ferketic, 1995). ASHA FACS represents an effort to specify key constructs of functional communicative disability in aphasia. The constructs selected were: (1) social communication, (2) communication of basic needs, (3) reading, writing, and number concepts, and (4) daily planning. Scoring of test items is accomplished through two separate scalings: a 7-point communicative independence ranking (quantitative) and a 5-point communicative dimensional ranking (qualitative). This test can be scored by either a clinician or a family member highly familiar with the patient's functional communicative abilities. All ASHA FACS behaviors reported here were scored by Hal.

c. **Well-being:** *Affect Balance Scale* (Bradburn, 1969). This standardized measure of well-being consists of 10 questions, half with positive and half with negative affect. These questions relate to general feelings about life, self, and others. Because it was not clear whether Betty's auditory and reading skills were sufficient to ensure full comprehension, Hal served as the respondent, attempting to represent Betty's perspective of her own well-being.

2. Nonstandardized Measures

a. **Communication:** *The Interactive Communication Scales.* A series of four interactive communicative scales, adapted from the qualitative portion of the ASHA FACS, was devised. Instead of ranking communication use in real-life according to its adequacy, appropriateness, promptness, or shared communicative burden, Hal was asked to rank its use according to comfort, confidence, connectedness, and pleasure. Table 9–1 describes each of these interactive dimensions and displays their 5-point ordinal ranking scale.

b. **Well-being:** *The Psychosocial Well-Being Index* (Lyon et al., 1997). The PWI was designed to capture change in the well-being of adults with aphasia as they participated in treatment aimed at increasing involvement in daily life. The test addresses four areas: general well-being; level of activity in daily life; feelings about self, family, or strangers; and comfort with self, family, or strangers. Scoring of target behaviors is along a 5-point ordinal scale. Hal did all pre- and post-treatment rankings of his perception of Betty's level of well-being.

Table 9–1. Interactive Communication Scales

Scale 1: Comfort

Definition: Degree of ease or comfort participants feel while interacting in spite of ongoing communicative limitations and/or failures in the exchange of information.

Very Uncomfortable   Uncomfortable   So...So   Comfortable   Very Comfortable

Scale 2: Confidence

Definition: Degree of confidence or assuredness that participants can resolve basic issues of daily life even when certain aspects of the exchange may remain unknown or confused due to communicative limitations.

Very Nonconfident   Nonconfident   So...So   Confident   Very Confident

Scale 3: Connectedness

Definition: Degree of connectedness or personally bonding that participants are able to maintain in spite of ongoing communicative limitations and/or failures in the exchange of information.

Very Unconnected   Unconnected   So...So   Connected   Very Connected

Scale 4: Pleasure

Definition: Degree of enjoyment or pleasure that participants find in interacting in spite of ongoing communicative limitations and/or failures in the exchange of information.

Very Unpleasant   Unpleasant   So...So   Pleasant   Very Pleasant

C. Results

A summary of pretreatment assessment results are in Table 9–2. In the area of language, Betty's overall BASA test score was severely depressed, placing her at the 16th percentile, compared with the standardized scores of other adults with severe and global aphasia. She was particularly impaired in auditory comprehension (5th percentile) and praxis (2nd percentile). ASHA FACS scores were commensurably depressed; only communication of basic needs appeared near a functional level of use (4.8 on a 7-point scale). ICS scores were the most deficient features of her communication, with only one scaled value above the lowest rating of 1, and it was a 2. ABS and PWI scores suggested that Betty's overall well-being was severely affected, as well.

Table 9-2. Pretreatment assessment of Hal and Betty

LANGUAGE: Standard and Percentile Scores from *Boston Assessment of Severe Aphasia* (Betty's test performance)

Subtest	Standard Score	Percentile Score
Auditory comprehension	5	5
Praxis	4	2
Oral-gestural expression	9	37
Reading comprehension	9	37
Other items	7	16
Overall	7	16

COMMUNICATION: ASHA *Functional Assessment of Communication Skills* (Hal's assessment of Betty)

Communication Independence Scores	Domain Mean (7–point ordinal scale)
Social communication (21 test items)	2.0
Communication of basic needs (7 test items)	4.8
Reading, writing, number concepts (10 test items)	1.8
Daily planning (5 test items)	1.6

Communication Qualitative Dimensions	Domain Mean (5–point ordinal scale)			
	Adequate	Appropr.	Prompt.	Comm. Sharing
Social communication	2.0	2.0	2	2
Communication of basic needs	3.0	3.0	3	3
Reading, writing, numbers	2.5	2.5	2	2
Daily planning	2.0	2.0	2	2

COMMUNICATION: *Interactive Communication Scales* (Hal's assessment of their abilities)

Interactive Communication Scales	Domain Mean (5–point ordinal scale)
Comfort	1
Confidence	1
Connectedness	2
Pleasure	1

WELL-BEING: *Affect Balance Scale and Psychosocial Well-Being Index* (Hal's assessment of Betty)

	Raw Score
Affect Balance Scale (10 test items) (dichotomous, yes/no scaling; 0–9 raw score)	1

	Mean Score
Psychosocial Well-being Index (11 test items) (5 point-ordinal scaling)	2.2

IV. DIAGNOSIS

A. The Disorder

I elected to type Betty's aphasia as severe. As measured on the BASA, her performance certainly fell within a "global classification." It is important to note, however, that Betty retained certain linguistic and nonlinguistic skills. For example, she had relatively good recognition of familiar, simple printed words and visual forms, pictures of famous figures from the past, numbers, and maps. Apraxia of speech may have been a concomitant factor, as there was notable oral groping when attempting to talk. Her BASA scores were suggestive of an oral, nonverbal apraxia as well. In any case, it was Betty's severe aphasia that presented this couple with their greatest communicative challenges and interfered the most with targeted treatment objectives.

B. Other Considerations

1. Changed Lifestyles

Betty's aphasia dramatically altered the daily life of both Hal and herself. Both had been highly independent and self-determined people before her stroke. Besides taking care of her grandchildren, Betty was an avid homemaker; baking bread daily, overseeing the upkeep of the house, and preparing all meals. In addition, she was a superb seamstress, making most of her grandchildren's clothes. Betty's aphasia and hemiplegia abruptly terminated all of these activities, ones that had given her life special meaning. Betty's problems terminated many of Hal's former activities, too, and entrapped him in a host of responsibilities, previously unknown or experienced.

2. Changed Roles

Betty's severe physical, social, communicative, and language dysfunctions all contributed to an ill-defined state of what was or was not possible in daily life. It is a state which Kagan (1995b) has referred to as one of "masked competencies," one in which lack of access to a viable communication system camouflages the underlying competency of a person with aphasia. This presumed incompetence is in the areas of cognitive and social ability that, without language, remain hidden from expression. The misperception of incompetence can be experienced by anyone who comes in direct contact with an injured party, including the patient, him or herself.

Although Kagan uses the "masked competencies" to refer to areas of cognitive and social competence, it can apply equally well to other realms of daily life, such as physical, psychological, and emotional. People with aphasia typically are capable of far more than they and others see as being possible. As a result, typically the more severe the aphasia, the more restricted one finds potential roles in daily life. Whereas many past functions may not be performed as completely, accurately, or efficiently as before, many are still "doable." Allowing people with aphasia to resume as much of living daily life as they might chose is the most "enabling" treatment we can provide. It is this "verifying process" of letting them act in their own behalf that establishes purpose and choice in daily life. It is these latter contingencies that I believe serve as the strongest catalysts in fostering and ensuring ongoing communication in natural settings.

When I met this couple, Betty had relinquished most of her prior daily duties in the home. Hal had assumed those responsibilities, as well as others for Betty's personal hygiene and daily care. Treatment, especially with respect to long-term objectives, was going to require an effort by both Hal and Betty to gradually shift some these daily responsibilities back to Betty.

V. PROGNOSIS

A. The Pros

The following factors spoke to a favorable outcome from therapy:

1. **Hal and Betty's Communication as a Couple Was a New Area to Explore.** Since her stroke, all treatment had focused on Betty's dysfunctional speech, language, or communication and never on their communication together. Hal and Betty were highly motivated to improve their communication as a couple and especially to learn strategies that might diminish their anguish in trying to cope with daily life.

2. **Betty Exhibited Linguistic and Nonlinguistic Strengthens That Might Aid Communication With Hal.** Her recognition of simple printed text was facilitative at certain times and under certain conditions. She was also aided by a variety of visual cues, such as pantomime or gesture, drawings, and maps. By combining these

approaches to communication, it was hypothesized that a more effective turn-taking interaction might occur.

3. **Both Parties Were Highly Disciplined,** dedicated to each other, and committed to any process that might improve their communication and lives. These qualities alone may not ensure therapeutic success, but without them, success is hard to orchestrate or predict.

B. The Cons

The following factors detracted from a favorable outcome to therapy:

1. **Betty was Extremely Sensitive to Any Failure on Her Part.** Whereas monitoring of one's own abilities is often perceived as a therapeutic asset, a high degree of self-criticism can be detrimental to treatment. There were occasions when Betty's inability to quickly grasp or perform a linguistic or communicative task immobilized any effort to move ahead. As a result, any simple stimulation task could begin as a warm, successful, interaction and abruptly stop with Betty in tears, unable to respond, and unwilling to proceed. For this treatment to work, some desensitization to occasional errors was necessary.

2. **Betty's Linguistic Level of Function was Highly Variable.** She experienced notable shifts in language/communication performance from hour-to-hour, day-to-day, and week-to-week. For a successful outcome, therapy required that such shifts be better understood and stabilized, if possible.

3. **Betty's Only Personal Power in Life was That Her Disabilities Kept Hal Nearby and Responding to Her Needs.** Betty had been successful homemaker and now performed few functions of housekeeping. Although she may have felt that her worth and value to Hal had diminished, she also may have sensed that her severely disabled condition kept him close at hand. If she grew more independent, she would not require as much of Hal's attention. This possibility could inadvertently subvert her efforts to seek greater independence.

4. **Hal and Betty had Established a "Dependency" Lifestyle.** Giving back responsibility for living life to a person with aphasia is infinitely more difficult when a dependency pattern has been established. The patient feels neglected, while the caregiver feels guilty.

For treatment to succeed, however, there must be a reversal of both feelings.

C. Expected Outcomes

The following outcomes were predicted for the first 3 months of treatment:

1. **Change in Language.** Little, if any, pre- or posttreatment change was expected on the overall BASA test scores and percentiles. The greatest changes on this measure were predicted to occur on the auditory and reading comprehension subtests, because of considerable treatment-related stimulation in the home setting.

2. **Change in Communication.** Moderate change was expected on portions of the ASHA FACS, especially those parts relating to social communication and communication of basic needs. More change was anticipated along quantitative rather than qualitative scales. This was because treatment emphasized the turn-taking with one another and not the adequacy, completeness, or proficiency of that exchange.

   The largest communicative change was expected where therapy was primarily focused: on ICS measures of comfort, confidence, connectedness, and pleasure. Beginning at levels near or at 1 on a 5-point scale, ICS values were expected to increase 2 to 4 scale points.

3. **Change in Well-being.** Some change in overall well-being was expected as a result of improved interactional communication skills between Betty and Hal. Larger gains, though, were predicted to follow after the treatment reported here, when long-term objectives could be targeted.

VI. TREATMENT

A. Introduction

1. The Period of Treatment

This section is an in-depth summary of the first section of treatment, extending from July 8, 1996 through September 28, 1996, and including 12 treatment sessions. The clinician met with Betty and Hal once weekly, and each treatment session lasted approximately

90 minutes. In this 3-month interim, only short-term objectives were addressed. However, the treatment process has continued, and long-term objectives are currently being addressed. As a result, the final segment of this section updates the current status of treatment.

2. The Nature of Treatment

The treatment described here involved eight treatment processes that were repeated during the 12 weeks this couple was seen. Table 9–3 displays a chronology of these eight steps and their functions throughout treatment. They are:

a. **Establishing a treatment target**—to specify a key target that would help merge Betty and Hal communicatively to further their success in interacting as a couple.

b. **Conceptualizing**—to formulate a plan for attaining the treatment target.

c. **Probing**—to investigate operative ways (often "transactional" in form) that might allow Betty and Hal to better interact.

d. **Demonstrating**—to allow the clinician to demonstrate to Betty and Hal how to use the proposed interactive format.

e. **Practicing**—to allow Hal and Betty to use the interactive methods while the clinician observed and assisted them.

f. **Implementing at home**—to design a plan for using the interactive methods at home.

g. **Functioning at home**—to assess the presence/absence and use/nonuse of interactive methods once implementation was attempted at home.

h. **Revising**—to modify interactive methods based on what had or had not worked at home.

Treatment, therefore, was a dynamic, cyclic process of targeting, conceiving, probing, practicing, implementing (at home), revising, retargeting, reconceiving, probing, practicing, implementing (at home), revising, and so on, until Betty and Hal merged as people communicating and working together in life.

Table 9–3 overviews six cyclic progressions in treatment, each involving eight steps aimed at bringing Betty and Hal closer as viable interactants in daily life. These steps were not rigidly prescribed. Instead, there was a freedom to modify the treatment form or methods based on whether use at home showed immediate signs of change or not. Such modifications relied primarily on this clinician's experiential knowledge of the intervening variables and what might enhance real-life use.

B. The Treatment Process

1. Cycle 1

The source of Hal and Betty's inability to interact effectively seemed to be twofold: (1) Hal's continuing assumption that Betty understood "almost everything he said," and (2) their inability to make use of Betty's existing communicative strengths. Given this scenario, treatment initially focused on demonstrating Betty's lack of comprehension and then on optimizing Betty's comprehension of Hal's spoken messages. This paradigm created a rudimentary transactional base from which to begin a communicative turn-taking process. It was also requisite to introducing other expressive means that Betty might use with Hal at home when she wished to share her own needs and wants.

As previously noted, both pantomime and printed cues appeared to facilitate Betty's comprehension of speech, although the severity of Betty's auditory comprehension deficit suggested that gestures alone might not suffice. Printed cues required more time to process, but they were more facilitative to Betty's comprehension and far more versatile (See Table 9–3, First Cycle, Probing). As a result, I began working toward a turn-taking exchange between Betty and me by simplifying verbal input, staying within a familiar communicative context (e.g., her children and grandchildren) and simultaneously printing key words of spoken messages. In this manner, Betty and I were able to exchange turns in a conversation about Hal and Betty's family. Hal observed this process and provided family members' names along the way. The clinician introduced a topic (e.g., "Which child is the oldest?"), using a printed list of names that provided Betty with a referent and a means by which to reply. She either pointed to a family member's name, requested additional information, or confirmed or disagreed with a clinician's suggested response.

Table 9–3. Treatment process displayed in steps and recurring cycles

Steps	First TX Cycle (2 weeks)	Second TX Cycle (2 weeks)	Third TX Cycle (2 weeks)
Treatment target	Increase this couple's ability to interact by increasing Hal's skill at using spoken messages that Betty would be mostly likely to understand.	Continue to build on current connectedness by re-emphasizing to Hal the fragility of Betty's comprehension of speech and the usefulness of print.	Continue to increase their interactive skills by examining Betty's comprehension abilities and limitations in using print.
Conceptualizing	As Betty's comprehension was increased by print and gesture on the BASA, their use should be probed.	Specifically contrast Betty's comprehension with and without printed cues with Hal observing.	Explore Betty's comprehension of printed cues in interaction outside familiar communicative contexts.
Probing	Pictured object identification (field of three) • auditory input: 15% • print input: 80% (delayed responses) • gesture input: 80%	Pictured object identification (field of three); began with just auditory, but in contrast to first probe, added print to each failed attempt; findings comparable to before but contrast impressive to Hal.	Comprehension of an unfamiliar topic probed using printed cues and a visually salient series of pictures; very difficult for Betty to do.
Demonstrating	Clinician talked to Betty about a familiar topic; key words printed out simultaneously on tablet between clinician and Betty; cues sequentially displayed midline of paper, top-to-bottom.	More specific demonstration of modifications to Hal's manner of interacting; fewer words spoken at a slower rate, writing key words legibly and in caps, and waiting for Betty to "verify" a point before moving on.	Demonstration to Hal that print may not be of value to Betty unless in familiar contexts; benefit depends on identifying the context first and then the content and keeping content basic.

Table 9–3. *(continued)*

Steps	First TX Cycle (2 weeks)	Second TX Cycle (2 weeks)	Third TX Cycle (2 weeks)
Practicing	Hal replicated clinician's use of printed aid; modifications made to his communicative style and use of print.	Hal showed increased success in interacting with Betty, particularly through his use of print.	Hal practiced interacting with Betty in some less familiar texts and tried to establish context and keep content simple.
Implementing at home	Tablets of paper distributed throughout house; Hal asked to support all verbal exchanges with printed cues.	Hal planned to supplement all important spoken messages to Betty by writing out key words.	Hal planned to use print at home only when Betty appeared puzzled; he gave context of the message first, verified that, then presented simple content.
Functioning at home	Minimal use (2–3 occasions per week); Hal considered writing "beneficial," but not all interactions successful; felt much better about interacting together.	Still minimal use (5–6 occasions per week); Hal reported that Betty was becoming resistant to his use of writing; even so, current method helped their overall "interactiveness" at home.	Use remained infrequent, but print far better received by Betty; still not always functional; Hal and Betty felt better as a couple about writing's use.
Revising	Hal indicated print usually not needed; Betty was familiar with most topics at home; clinician decided to demonstrate further evidence of print's usefulness.	Clinician decided to address Betty's reasons for not wanting to use printed cues.	Clinician felt more successful in finding a functional system for Betty and Hal; print proved helpful only if it was presented at the right time and in the right form.

Table 9–3. *(continued)*

Steps	Fourth TX Cycle (2 weeks)	Fifth TX Cycle (2 weeks)	Sixth TX Cycle (2 weeks)
Treatment target	Fine tune Betty and Hal's interactive skills through "selective" use of print and improving ways of understanding Hal's speech.	Search for an interactive way that Betty might reliably "share" basic needs and wants with Hal at home.	Find a more functional way that Betty might share needs with Hal at home, while preserving her expression of communicative intent.
Conceptualizing	Examine further ways of maximizing Betty's comprehension of Hal's speech.	Given Betty's recognition of simple, common printed/pictured stimuli, probe their use as an expressive aid; success already known in printed breakfast menu of options.	Betty often sat in one room of the house and pointed toward somewhere else; Hal responded through probes and fetching possible items; explore a functional probe.
Probing	Pictured object identification (field of three) with auditory input; speaker facing Betty, awaiting her signal to proceed, "alerting" her to on-coming stimulus; 15% accuracy without aids and 60–70% with; 85% accuracy when function of object added.	Recognition and identification of printed words in functional lists: important people, places, things, and activities at home; Betty's skill not as reliable as with breakfast menu (only 30–60% accuracy); shifted to taking pictures of items to supplement print.	Use of floor plans or home maps to help identify needs; also, began urging more active role on Betty's part, such as, having her take Hal to requested items/locations in house; her physical capabilities didn't permit this at first but now do.
Demonstrating	Demonstration of picture identification task as a model for Hal to use at home.	Demonstration of picture/print identification task using commonly requested items at home.	Demonstrate use of floor plans to indicate where common objects were in the house and where to go to meet various needs.

Table 9–3. (continued)

Steps	Fourth TX Cycle (2 weeks)	Fifth TX Cycle (2 weeks)	Sixth TX Cycle (2 weeks)
Practicing	Hal practiced task, replicating clinician's pace and manner; provided printed word, if needed.	Hal practiced same task with Betty while clinician observed.	Hal asked Betty where other common items were.
Implementing at home	Hal and Betty interacted at home each day using the strategies practiced in the clinic (See Table 9–4).	Hal, Betty, and clinician located a central place at home where pictures/printed stimuli might be easily displayed and assessed, on kitchen refrigerator.	Betty was provided a floor plan to use when requesting at home; if Hal was not able to discern an item after a single attempt, he urged her to go there.
Functioning at home	Hal reported "much improved" interactive process at home; used "some" writing but less; adapted his speech more to form and style used in picture identification task.	None; Betty had agreed to proposed task in clinic but resisted display of these stimuli at home; resistance seemed related to lack of clarity about their use.	Betty was openly agreeable to plan and used it successfully several times; Betty was willing to show Hal a location when the plan did not work.
Revising	Although clinician saw that speech and cueing strategies were becoming comfortable and used in home, the prime breakdown now was in Hal's understanding Betty's needs.	Clinician hypothesized a problem of representation, a lack of saliency of the stimuli at the time of expressive need; Betty required output with stronger bond between intent and means of expression.	Building on a successful system for requests "in-house," the clinician next envisioned an interactive means that might aid Betty's requests outside the home.

From a distance, this form of interacting might not appear all that different from traditional treatments aimed at transacting information. Certainly, the ongoing process between Betty and me seemed to be an exchange of information about family members. However, procuring information about Hal and Betty's family was not the therapeutic intent. Instead, the intent was to engage in a process that enabled Betty to be an equal interactant with me. Betty's transactional responses were not minimized as we uncovered information about her family tree. The "tree" was just a topic, but one that allowed interaction to happen. A shared topic of interest was needed to move this turn-taking process forward, but whether or not these conversational "turns" were accurate or complete did not matter. It was valuable to demonstrate this distinction to Hal, and to let him see first hand that getting Betty's participation in the exchange was far more important to our mutual enjoyment than whether I had understood all the subtleties about family members. Such a demonstration allowed Hal to rethink his own insistence on the accuracy of shared content and to shift his attention instead to interacting. My sole treatment goals at first were to enable Betty to feel successful again as a communicator, someone who is valued as a viable interactant in a turn-taking process, and to give Hal a new definition of a successful interaction.

Once a viable transactional and interactional system was in place, Hal and the clinician shifted roles; Hal became the interactant with Betty with the clinician becoming the observer. Hal's natural speech was faster than the clinician's and contained many descriptors and qualifiers. The volume of information he tried to share quickly confused Betty. Hal's writing was also more rapid and, on certain occasions, was illegible to her. Over the next several weeks at the clinic, we worked as a communicative team toward modifying Hal's timing and inputs with Betty in turn-taking exchanges.

After Hal felt comfortable interacting with Betty in the clinic, he distributed paper and pens throughout the house and began supplementing his spoken messages with written key words. To assess the usefulness of writing, Hal was asked to bring their written supplements to conversation to weekly sessions. At first, the number of supported interactions at home was far below expected levels. Hal only used writing on two or three occasions the first week, a number anticipated to occur within the first hour of the first day. When questioned about this, Hal maintained that Betty understood his spoken messages in this environment and there was little need to write out key words. He maintained that as Betty knew their setting and their daily routine, her comprehension was sufficient in most interactions without written cueing.

2. Cycle 2

Although I was convinced of Betty's dire need for printed cueing to remain interactive with me in the clinic, it seemed that Hal was still not fully cognizant of Betty's limited auditory comprehension skills. To illustrate her need, I elected to reprobe Betty's ability to respond to an auditory picture identification task without and with written cues. Initially, auditory stimuli were given and repeated several times. When Betty appeared confused or unwilling to respond, which typically was the case, a written stimulus was added. Betty's common reaction to the printed cue was a slightly delayed but accurate response, allowing Hal to once again see the communicative value of this aid.

By week 4 of treatment, more writing was occurring at home (increasing from 2–3 occurrences weekly to 5–7 occurrences), but levels of use remained far below what I had anticipated. Now, for the first time, Hal reported that Betty was beginning to reject his attempts to use written cues at home. This resistance seemed to stem more from Betty's perception of the worth of this aid than from Hal's manner of use. It appeared that some topics Hal tried to introduce were more confusing with writing than without.

3. Cycle 3

As a result of Betty's rejection of Hal's written cues, the functionality and versatility of printed cues at home fell into question. Instead of the familiar topics and stimuli of previous weeks, I decided to probe supplemental writing in a less familiar context, yet one that was accessible through pictured stimuli (e.g., showing Betty a thematic scene from *Life* magazine in which a woman is rescued from a stranded car in a flooding river). Despite returning to the same turn-taking techniques from our earlier conversations, Betty quickly became lost in this task. Once confused, she ceased to participate and withdrew. Not only was the turn-taking process interrupted, but she displayed dismay, and even tears over her seeming inability to stay with the task. I was unable to return her to a participatory level even by trying to bolster her viability as a turn-taker through the use of other "total communication" strategies.

It appeared as if Betty's withdrawal from this task was due to its inherent complexity and her keen sensitivity to not responding at what she considered an acceptable level. As confirmation of this, she instantly resumed a participatory role as a turn-taker a week later, when the content and context were once again shifted back to a familiar, simplified, and well-supported theme. Any attempt to move toward a less familiar context resulted in Betty's return to the behavior of the previous week. The bottom line seemed to be that Betty preferred tolerating some misunderstanding of Hal's spoken messages at home to succumbing to the confusion and discouragement of deciphering Hal's printed cues in an unfamiliar context. What I had learned was that for an interaction to work, Betty required transactional success when a nonstandard mode of writing was used. When the transactional load exceeded her comfort level, all interaction ceased. Thus, I either needed to keep writing within an acceptable level of use or work on enhancing the more standard mode of spoken input.

4. Cycle 4

Because of the restricted use of writing at home, I began looking for other ways of increasing Hal and Betty's turn-taking capabilities in that environment. If Betty preferred Hal's spoken words alone to those supplemented by writing, it was then crucial to determine how we might maximize her comprehension of these messages. Additional probes were readied using the prior picture identification task. Now I positioned myself directly across from her, allowed her to control the rate of presentation and alerted her to the forthcoming stimuli. If confused or unable to respond, Betty was given several associative features about the stimulus. If Betty was still stymied, I wrote out the stimulus for her.

Not only was Betty's auditory comprehension improved (from 15% without these speaker-related adjustments to 85% with them and 100% when the printed cue was added), it provided an excellent interactional framework for the couple to practice at home. That is, Hal first awaited Betty's signal that she was ready to interact. He consciously altered his verbal output, first by alerting her to forthcoming content and then by keeping that content simple and concise. This procedure also allowed him to notice and to solicit a turn-taking response from her. Finally, it allowed for a communicative context in which print did aid both participants. Through this transactional task, they practiced and perfected their interactive skills at home.

What evolved from this clinically based task to the home setting was a turn-taking procedure that Hal and Betty could modify to improve their communication in daily life. Table 9–4 details the specific communicative strategies that permitted Hal and Betty to interact more comfortably and freely in daily life. From these, Hal reported increased confidence in his ability to structure his spoken

Table 9–4. Communication suggestions for Hal for interacting with Betty

General Recommendations

1. Always directly face her
   - This allows her to see you
   - More importantly, it allows you to see her.

2. Present your points **concisely** and **one-at-a-time.**

3. Look for a "confirming" nod or word from her (e.g., okay, yes, o' boy)
   - If it's **decisive** and **quick,** it usually means...she has it
   - If its **slow** or equivocal, it usually means...something is **not** clear.

4. Constantly reverify when Betty has been successful.

5. Enjoy yourself!

How To Aid Her When Her Response Is Not Decisive Or Quick

1. Make your point again
   - State it in a slightly different way, but still trying to keep it clear and concise.

2. Write out in "BIG CAPS" the word or phrase in question
   - De-emphasize the writing
   - Don't announce or talk about it...make it a natural EXTENSION of conversation
     for example: "oops...something is not quite right...take a look at this"
   - Back further up
     *Provide more CONTEXT
     *Keep it simple
       for example: "I'm talking about...**dinner**...**tonight."**
         (bold words written out)
       restate earlier point..."Do you want a **potato**?"

SUMMARY

1. Focus on "staying connected," NOT on the tools (e.g., writing).

2. Always gauge your response based on hers!!!
   - move ahead when she has clearly understood and is with you.
   - back up and try to AID her when she isn't understood.

3. **Keep your communication aids in the background of interacting**
   - They are secondary to staying connected
   - If they become the "main part" of the exchange, they often hamper rather than facilitate.

message so Betty could respond, and, together, they began pursuing and attaining resolutions on topics previously ignored or had often created confusion. For Hal, what remained most problematic in the interactions, though, was how to discern Betty's basic needs and wants.

5. Cycle 5

To aid this couple in establishing turn-taking attempts at addressing Betty's needs, one practical option seemed to be printed lists. One such list, a list of breakfast choices, had already proven successful in allowing Betty to specify her daily preferences. So, I next compiled lists of people, events, places, and other things that might also aid the pair's interactions. The use of these lists, even in the clinic, however, proved too challenging for Betty. Many of stimuli seemed too complex, and, somehow, their presence within the home seemed to interfere with her own communicative intent.

Photographs were next probed as communication aids, with no better results. In fact, Betty simply refused to have these pictured stimuli displayed in any readily accessible place or manner in the home. This refusal did not seem to emanate from a rejection of the task; that is, it was not because she did not want to seek any alternative way that she and Hal might interact communicatively. Instead, it seemed that pictures simply failed to adequately capture the entirety of what she wished to communicate. For example, a picture/printed word of a desired item could be positioned right next to her, and she would opt instead to point toward the item's location within the house, even if this was four rooms removed. Although pictures and printed words seemed a logical adjunct to Hal and me, they did not to Betty!

6. Cycle 6

As Betty rejected any use of pictured/printed symbols in the home and instead tended toward directional pointing, I next probed the use of house maps. Floor plans of the entire house were drawn, with designations for the main pieces of furniture, appliances, and objects. Probes were designed to assess her ability and willingness to indicate wants and desires using this graphic aid. Betty readily and enthusiastically responded, in contrast to the probes undertaken in Cycle 5.

With minimal practice in the clinic, Hal and Betty began using this visual aid at home. Hal immediately reported several occasions during which Betty had successfully indicated a need via the house maps. Also, when the plan was not available or adequate, Betty was willing, for the first time, to physically get up and take Hal to the desired item. At the end of the 132nd week of therapy, I was able to begin extending the use of maps to places outside the home where Betty could communicate her needs and wants.

C. Treatment Follow Up

Two months have passed since the above treatment period ended. In that interim, therapy has continued. Here is a brief update on Hal and Betty's progress:

1. Short-Term Objectives

Initial steps have been taken to find ways for Betty to communicate about topics outside the home. Again, visually oriented stimuli have proven the most effective. Neighborhood, city, state, and national maps are frequently referenced. Also, pictures of key people, places, and activities have begun to enhance the couple's exchanges. Whereas Betty was resistant to using pictures of objects within the home, she now readily relies on pictures of people or places outside the home. In addition, Betty and Hal are interactively taking turns in referring to printed, familiar lists when that content and context are well-defined and match Betty's communicative intent. Hal and Betty are reporting that they are interactively satisfying each other's needs on a daily basis. Neither person indicates an unwillingness, uncomfortableness, or inability to attend to the other in a time of need. There has been an obvious merging in their interactions as a couple over time. Basically, they appear to have reached an amicable means of connecting with one another, regardless of whether or not their message has been fully understood or heeded.

2. Long-Term Objectives

Probes have begun, with the goal of finding ways for Hal and Betty to assume greater independence in daily life. For example, Betty now has a secure means of summoning Hal at any time he is away from the house (via a programmed phone at home and a cellular phone with Hal). With Betty having this security, Hal has begun leaving their home for short durations. Not only does this allow him to attend to outside responsibilities, but it sets the stage for Betty to begin assuming more responsibility for herself.

In addition, Betty has begun several former pursuits from her pre-stroke days. After baking her first batch of cookies with Hal's assistance, she has just completed her first cross-stitch embroidery project. Although she will point out that it is not perfect (she has always been a perfectionist), this accomplishment has notably enhanced her self-esteem and pride. She will begin another pattern next week. Also, she is currently looking through seed catalogs and planning this year's flower garden, although planting remains a couple of months away.

VII. RESULTS

Treatment results are summarized in Table 9–5.

A. Language

Several language-related domains on the BASA showed marked improvement or decline. Those improving were: auditory comprehension, with percentile score change from 5 to 25; reading comprehension, with a percentile shift from 25 to 50; and other items, with percentile levels increasing from 25 to 50. Oral-gestural expression declined, with a percentile change from 37 to 16, secondary to Betty's perseverative block across all verbal imitation test items.

Percentile differences reflected standard scores, a standard score change of more than two points pre-, posttreatment represented a statistically significant improvement or decline.

B. Communication

Despite what had been predicted, Betty improved on all ASHA FACS communication independence scores. On a 7-point scale, mean scores increased about one scale point, with communication of basic needs changing the most. Qualitative dimensions on the ASHA FACS changed little, perhaps reflective of the minimal emphasis placed on these realms in treatment. The key focus of treatment, interactive communication, substantially increased on ICS measures, noting 1- to 2-point gains across all realms: comfort, confidence, connectedness, and pleasure.

C. Well-Being

Overall well-being measures showed little change over the initial 13-week period of treatment (ABS score increased by 2 points on a 10-point

Table 9–5. Comparison of pre-, posttreatment assessments of Hal and Betty

LANGUAGE: Standard and Percentile Scores from *Boston Assessment of Severe Aphasia* (Betty's test performance)

Subtest	Pretreatment		Posttreatment		Difference	
	Std Score	% Score	Std Score	% Score	Std Score	% Score
Auditory comprehension	5	5	8	25	+3	+20
Praxis	4	2	4	2	0	0
Oral-gestural expression	9	37	7	16	−2	−21
Reading comprehension	9	37	11	63	+2	+26
Other items	7	16	10	50	+3	+25
OVERALL	7	16	8	21	+1	+5

COMMUNICATION: ASHA *Functional Assessment of Communication Skills* (Hal's assessment of Betty)

Communication Independence Scores

	Domain Mean (7–point ordinal scale)		
	Pre-tx	Post-tx	Difference
Social communication (21 test items)	2.0	2.7	+0.7
Communication of basic needs (7 test items)	4.8	6.1	+1.3
Reading, writing, number concepts (10 test items)	1.8	2.1	I 0.3
Daily planning (5 test items)	1.6	2.4	+0.8

Communication Qualitative Dimensions	Domain Mean (5–point ordinal scale)											
	Adequate			Appropr.			Prompt.			Comm. Sharing		
	PRE	POST	DIFF	PRE	POST	DIFF	PRE	POST	DIFF	PRE	POST	DIFF
Social communication	2.0	2.0	0	2.0	2.0	0	2.0	2.5	+.5	2	2	0
Communication of basic needs	3.0	3.0	0	3.0	3.0	0	3.0	3.0	0.0	3	3	0
Reading, writing, numbers	2.5	2.5	0	2.5	2.5	0	2.0	2.0	0.0	2	2	0
Daily planning	2.0	2.0	0	2.0	2.0	0	2.0	2.0	0.0	2	2	0

Interactive Communication Scales (Hal's assessment of their abilities)

Interactive Communication Scales	Domain Mean (5–point ordinal scale)		
	Pretreatment	Posttreatment	Difference
Comfort	1	2.5	+1.5
Confidence	1	3.0	+2.0
Connectedness	2	3.0	+1.0
Pleasure	1	3.0	+2.0

WELL-BEING: Raw Score Differences from *Affect Balance Scale* (Hal's assessment of Betty)

Pretreatment	Posttreatment	Difference
1	3	+2

Mean Score Differences from the Psychosocial Well-Being Index

Pretreatment	Posttreatment	Difference
2.2	2.2	0

scale, with the mean PWI score unchanged). Although Hal and Betty were beginning to establish better ways of interacting, changes in daily life had not yet mirrored these gains. Two months later, however, Hal and Betty are reporting increased independence or freedom in both of their daily routines.

VIII. DISCUSSION

A. Was This Treatment of Value?

Managed care now mandates that we focus treatment on improving functional use of communicative skills. However, the optimal time and methods for accomplishing these ends remain unclear. In reporting my therapy with this couple, I have tried to illustrate that treatment at home entails developing the interactional as well as the transactional components of communication. Success may depend, as well, on showing, coaching, and revising methods of turn-taking within the treated couple's personal interactive repertoires at home. The outcomes derived here suggest that merging patient and caregiver in terms of their comfort, confidence, connectedness, and pleasure in interacting may be requisite to providing better and lasting communicative use in natural settings. These data, however, neither address nor attempt to prove the efficacy of this treatment. Very simply, they point to an approach not reported as a part of past treatments, that may prove important in establishing communicative use in real life.

B. Other Alternatives to This Treatment

There probably are many ways of improving functional use of communication in daily life; many are needed, and more are beginning to surface. Kagan (1995a) has described the value of community-based centers to increase communicative access to participation in various aspects of social and community life. Hinckley, Packard, and Bardach (1995) have emphasized the use of a university residential care center to foster family educational needs. Ford, Walker-Batson, and Curtis (1995) have documented the development of a university-based aphasia center model that provides ongoing graduate student training, while permitting people with chronic aphasia and their caregivers to become more functionally "enabled" in daily life. Simpson (1989), Marshall (1993), Kagan and Gailey (1993), Beeson and Holland (1994), and Elman and Bernstein-Ellis (1996) have fostered differing ways of using aphasia peer-group interaction to improve conversational and social skills in daily life. Lyon et al. (1997) has enlisted community volunteers to help move adults with aphasia out into their respective societies with more independent and self-sustaining lifestyles. In Great Britain, the member-supported Action for Dysphasic Adults enables adults with aphasia to set group agendas in their own behalf (ADA, 1994). Thus, treatment options for effecting change in communication in natural settings are just beginning to evolve.

C. Hindsights

It is possible that the treatment described here could have evolved more directly than it did. As it was, I began with printed cues to augment Betty's severely impaired auditory comprehension, only to "learn" weeks later that their successful use at home relied on a highly familiar verbal context. In the end, printed words were abandoned in favor of more simplified spoken messages. Such adjustments should not be viewed as "errors." They are, in fact, integral and essential parts of this treatment process. Finding effective and enduring strategies that satisfy what might and will work in everyday life is not bound to any known "clinical prescription." To date, such prescriptions have yet to show effective transfer to natural settings. A successful process depends, instead, on a dynamic interplay between therapist and treated parties in both clinical and real-life settings. Only when a collective blend emerges from what is possible, and then what is preferrable, is a lasting solution apt to evolve. It is this process of searching out the operative and salient variables for interactants that is most needed. These variables are linked to the treated individuals, their communicative needs, and their communicative contexts. With time and greater experience in differentiating these factors, clinicians will be better able to surmise which treatment options are most universal in application and which are idiosyncratic.

D. What This All Means

There are many treatment options awaiting exploration that might improve functional communication for people with severe aphasia. Because many of these options rest out there in the "real world" with all its complexities, they may appear too complicated at times to undertake. Quite likely, their prime variables are ill-defined and unlikely to fit neatly into an either-or scenario. Such was the case here. Fixing communication is not about "interacting" versus "transacting" or about "transacting" versus "interacting." Both components are essential to the integrity of the whole. One must have joint access to and interest in a topic to converse, but the accuracy of information shared is a small part of the rich story of friendship and caring. By finding and better defining of the proper mix between these components, we may move closer to restoring functional communication in the daily lives of the people we treat.

IX. REFERENCES

Action for Dysaphasic Adults (1994). *Unlocking words: Annual report '94.* London: Author.

Beeson, P., & Holland, A. (1994). *Aphasia groups: An approach to long-term rehabilitation (Telerounds #19).* Tucson, AZ: National Center for Neurogenic Communication Disorders.

Bradburn, N. M. (1969). *The structure of psychological well-being.* Chicago: Aldine.

Elman, R., & Bernstein-Ellis, E. (1995). What is functional? *American Journal of Speech-Language Pathology, 4*(4), 115–117.

Elman, R., & Bernstein-Ellis, E. (1996, June). *Effectiveness of group communication treatment for individuals with chronic aphasia: Results on communicative and linguistic measures.* Paper presented at Clinical Aphasiology Conference, Newport, RI.

Ford, J., Walker-Batson, D. & Curtis, S. (1995, November). *A transdisciplinary approach to long-term aphasia rehabilitation.* Miniseminar presented at annual convention of the American Speech-Language-Hearing Association, Orlando, FL.

Frattali, C. (1996, December). Measuring disability: The garian group. In R. Warren (Ed.), *Neurophysiology and Neurogenic Speech and Language Disorders Special Interest Division 2 Newsletter,* (pp. 7–10) Rockville, MD: American Speech-Language Hearing Association.

Frattali, C. M., Thompson, C. K., Holland, A. L., Wohl, C. B., & Ferketic, M. M. (1995). *American Speech-Language-Hearing Association: Functional assessment of communicative skills.* Rockville, MD: American Speech-Language-Hearing Association.

Helm-Estabrooks, N., Ramsberger, G., Morgan, A. R, & Nicholas, M. (1989). *Boston Assessment of Severe Aphasia.* Chicago: Applied Symbolix.

Hinckley, J. J., Packard, M. E. W., & Bardach, L. G. (1995). Alternative family education programming for adults with chronic aphasia. *Topics in Stroke Rehabilitation, 2*(3), 53–63.

Holland, A. L. (1992). Some thoughts on future needs and directions for research and treatment of aphasia. *NIDCD Monograph, 2,* 147–152.

Kagan, A. (1995a). Family perspectives from three aphasia centers in Ontario, Canada. *Topics in Stroke Rehabilitation, 2*(3), 1–19.

Kagan, A. (1995b). Revealing the competence of aphasic adults through conversation: A challenge to health professionals. *Topics in Stroke Rehabilitation, 2*(1), 15–28.

Kagan, A., & Gailey, G. F. (1993). Functional is not enough: Training conversation partners for aphasic adults. In A. L. Holland & M. M. Forbes (Eds.), *Aphasia Treatment: World Perspectives* (pp. 199–225). San Diego, CA: Singular Publishing Group, Inc.

Lyon, J. G. (1992). Communication use and participation in life for adults with aphasia in natural settings: The scope of the problem. *American Journal of Speech-Language Pathology, 1*(3), 7–14.

Lyon, J. G. (1996, December). Measurement of treatment effects in natural settings. In R. Warren (Ed.), *Neurophysiology and Neurogenic Speech and Language*

Disorders Special Interest Division 2 Newsletter, (pp. 10–15) Rockville, MD: American Speech-Language-Hearing Association.

Lyon, J. G., Cariski, D., Keisler, L., Rosenbek, J., Levine, R., Kumpula, J., Ryff, C., Coyne, S., & Blanc, M. (1997). Communication partners: Enhancing participation in life and communication for adults with aphasia in natural settings. *Aphasiology, 11*(7), 693–708.

Marshall, R. C. (1993). Problem-focused group treatment for clients with mild aphasia. *American Journal of Speech-Language Pathology, 2,* 31–37.

Simmons N. (1993). *An ethnographic investigation of compensatory strategies in aphasia.* Unpublished doctoral dissertation, Louisiana State University: Baton Rouge.

Simmons-Mackie, N., & Damico, J. S. (in press). Accounting for handicaps in aphasia: Communicative assessment from an authentic social perspective. *Disability and Rehabilitation.*

Simpson, M. (1989, September). Stroke support and stroke family groups: An adjunct to generalization. Presentation at the Speech and Stroke Centre in North York, Ontario, Canada.

Warren, R. (1996, December). Outcomes measurement: Moving toward the patient. In R. Warren (Ed.), *Neurophysiology and Neurogenic Speech and Language Disorders Special Interest Division 2 Newsletter,* (pp. 5–6). Rockville, MD: American Speech-Language-Hearing Association.

World Health Organization (1980). *International classification of impairments, disabilities, and handicaps.* Geneva, Switzerland: Author.

CHAPTER

10

Clinical Care in a Changing Health System

CAROL M. FRATTALI, Ph.D.

"It's not a perfect world—people are making up answers to questions based on economics and not efficacy. Our goal is to come to some agreement between the two."

—Robert T. Wertz, 1996

I. INTRODUCTION

Health care is being redefined and restructured aggressively to control its spiraling costs. Byproducts of the change include staff reductions, treatment limits, and lower cost alternatives to traditional care. These and other cost-cutting measures will only become more common as various managed care models proliferate and as federally mandated projects develop prospective payment methodologies for medical rehabilitation. Soon, traditional models of clinical practice may become obsolete. Delivery of care will require a balance of quality care with the bottom line, that is, alignment of clinical service with the concept of *value* (good outcomes at a low cost) for health care dollars spent.

In this chapter I take a "purse-strings" approach to aphasia treatment and look beyond traditional models of clinical practice and clinical research. This is a good time to reframe our thinking and restructure our treatments to create cost-effective and beneficial programs that are meaningful to patients, their families, and those paying the bills. To those who believe that this approach is payer- rather than provider-driven, I would suggest that it is neither. It puts the consumer at the helm of the system—an approach that has been shaped by several influences.

A. Influences Shaping a Consumer-Directed Approach to Care

1. **A Social Definition of Quality Care.** As clinicians, I believe that we are responsible not just for our individual patients, but for the patient population at-large (i.e., the entire pool of candidates in current or future need of our services). Thus, in a system of finite resources, the excessive or unnecessary care we provide to one patient may deny another the most basic care. According to Donabedian (1980), the highest quality of care is that which yields the highest net utility for the entire population in need of that care. Donabedian states further that, "the use of redundant care, even when it is harmless, indicates carelessness, poor judgment, or ignorance on the part of the practitioner who is responsible for care. It contravenes the rule of 'parsimony,' which has been, traditionally, the hallmark of virtuosity in clinical performance" (p. 7). In plainer terms, excessive care in today's health care climate violates the ethical boundaries of any clinical field. It ignores the concept of value, which should characterize our treatments.

2. **Increased Specialization in Health Care.** Medical specialization is fragmenting service and adding to the complexity and cost of care. Although this specialization is a natural byproduct of the expansion of scientific and clinical knowledge, its casualty often is the patient who suffers from a lack of a coordinated or holistic approach to care or is denied access to specialized care because of its expense.

3. **Regulatory Reforms.** In several cases, regulatory reforms (e.g., accreditation standards of the Joint Commission on Accreditation

of Health Care Organizations, Medicare Conditions of Participation) have removed requirements of certification from specific professional associations and instituted clinical competencies as prime indicators of clinician qualifications. Letters after clinicians' names are no longer considered proof of skills. Instead, clinicians must both define and document their competencies to accreditation agencies and payers. In some cases where clinicians are not meeting this requirement, these outside agents or the medical staff of the facilities in which clinicians work are defining clinician competencies and enforcing these standards.

4. **Lack of Convincing Treatment Data.** Our field has yet to provide legislators, regulators, and payers with convincing proof of general treatment efficacy or effectiveness or to demonstrate that lower cost alternatives to treatment produce less desirable outcomes. Furthermore, from both clinical and economic points of view, it is not enough to know whether treatment works; it must be determined whether one treatment works better than another for a particular disorder.

5. **Emerging Models of Care.** The traditional focus of treatment has been remediation of specific skills rather than enhancement of a person's ability to adjust to residual problems. In either case, one must ask whether improvements in patients' functions have consequences for their quality of life—are they worth the time, effort, and money spent? New models based on an integration of social science (e.g., the patient's perception of health, functional status, quality of life) rather than medical science paradigms (diagnosis and cure) are just recently gaining the attention of the health care community and are predicted to influence approaches to service delivery.

6. **Consumer Choice and Satisfaction.** As consumers become more knowledgeable and active in decisions that affect their lives, they are exercising their options to choose from among several health plan offerings and to change plans if they are not satisfied. Thus, consumer satisfaction becomes an important outcome of care, not only for the consumer but for the health plan with economic interest in retaining enrollees.

Now I will describe salient features of our changing health care system, determine how some of the case studies contained in this volume might fit within such a system, and discuss what the case studies are teaching us and how this knowledge might be used. Finally, I will offer some recommendations that might serve us in the near and distant future as we continue to treat patients with aphasia.

II. THE CHANGING HEALTH CARE SYSTEM

It is predicted that by the year 2000 all health care will be managed in one form or another. Although we need to prepare for federally mandated changes, the most pervasive changes will be market-driven. The growth of managed care plans, including health maintenance organizations (HMOs), preferred provider organizations (PPOs), and independent practice associations (IPAs), represents the impetus for forcible changing of the "where's," "how's," and "how long's" of patient care. Patients are being discharged "quicker and sicker" from acute care hospitals, giving rise to a new level of care called "subacute," to denote its position between acute care and nursing facility care.

Short hospital stays have accelerated the growth of industries such as nursing facilities, home health, and outpatient care. Cost cutting has resulted in caps on services and limits on number of sessions, length of treatment, and level of reimbursement. As a result, patient evaluation and treatment plans must be modified. Given these constraints, we must decide how to best use the shrinking resources for providing quality care. To make these decisions, we must understand the changing health care system.

A. Managed Care

The most sweeping changes in health care involve managed care in all its hybrid forms. Generally, managed care describes a cost-effective system that integrates both the financing and delivery of health care services. It is defined by the American Association of Health Plans (American Managed Care and Review Association, 1995), the national trade association representing managed care organizations, as a comprehensive approach to health care delivery that encompasses planning and coordination of care, patient and provider education, monitoring of care quality, and cost control.

In the 1980s, at the crest of the "health care crisis" in America, managed care was considered an answer to spiraling costs and the secrecy that seemed to surround medical care and its clinical and financial effectiveness. Today's critics say that managed care neither manages nor cares and that the only interest is the dollar saved. Clearly, cost is of prime interest to managed care administrators. Cost consciousness, however, is not necessarily bad when it is accompanied by an ethical sense of decision making and honest yardsticks against which to measure the goodness of patient care.

1. **Common Care Management Features.** Three features of care management are important to clinicians: *gatekeeper functions, utilization review or management,* and *treatment authorization.* A *gatekeeper* is the coordinator of a patient's care. The gatekeeper approach requires the patient to gain access to the entire system of care through a single, experienced primary care physician. Thus, the gatekeeper decides what care the patient needs and usually at what intensity and scope of service. *Utilization review/management* (UR) (recently being called *resource management*) is a systematic process of reviewing and controlling patients' use of health care services and providers' use of health care resources. UR procedures include second opinions, precertifications, treatment authorizations, discharge planning, and chart reviews. Finally, *authorization* is approval for care or services. These features create a system of checks and balances designed to prevent unnecessary, inappropriate, or excessive care and ensure the quality of care. In effect, they lead to compliance with the regulations for rehabilitative services imposed by Congress for federally qualified HMOs. The Federal HMO Act of 1973 states:

   Federally qualified HMOs must provide or arrange for outpatient service and inpatient hospital services which shall include short-term rehabilitation and physical therapy, the provision of which the HMO determines can be expected to result in the significant improvement of a member's condition within a period of two months. (Code of Federal Regulations, Title 42, Section 110.102[1990])

   The emphasis here is on "short-term." Although 2 months was specified in the regulatory language as a minimum time period of treatment, it often is interpreted by managed care administrators as a maximum. In all, the language of the federal law carries great significance for clinicians whose usual ways of providing care extend well beyond this time period.

2. **Common Forms of Payment.** The two common forms of payment to practitioners who work in managed care contexts are *discounted fee-for-service* and *capitation. Discounted fee-for-service* is a discount from the provider's usual or customary fee, paid after services are rendered. As a cost-containment strategy, this option has failed. To offset the impact of the discounts, providers have increased usual

rates or increased the frequency and types of services. *Capitation* is a fixed amount of money set by contract between a managed care organization (MCO) and the provider, to be paid on a per-person (per capita) basis regardless of the number of services rendered or costs incurred. Capitation is usually expressed in cost units of "per member per month (PMPM)." Typically, the MCO sets aside a percentage of the payment to safeguard against unexpected costs. At the year's end, any money left in this risk pool is returned to the providers. Capitation is a shared risk arrangement, which provides incentives for physicians (often the gatekeepers of care) to limit special tests, special services (including rehabilitation), and hospitalization for the enrollees. The scope of services in a capitation contract can range from limited primary care physician services to all health care services. As providers are expected to share more risk, the primary payment arrangement is shifting to capitation.

Fee-for-service gives caregivers little or no financial incentive to be concerned about the cost and use (or overuse) of services. Thus, to earn more money, the incentive is to increase utilization. This payment arrangement rewards piecework; the more services providers render, the more money they make. Conversely, *capitation* fundamentally changes the financial incentives of traditional fee-for-service systems because it is a fixed revenue system that pays the same amount each month no matter how many or how few services are actually provided. Effectively, the fewer services provided, the more the providers are rewarded. Under capitation, the provider's primary objective is to maximize quality of care and patient satisfaction and minimize the total cost of care per person per year. *Value* (good quality at a low cost), then, becomes the primary demand of major purchasers of health care (e.g., employers) and consumers.

3. **Typical Managed Care Coverage Limitations.** For speech-language pathology and other rehabilitative services, managed care organizations may impose one or more resictions and limit services to:

- 60 days

- 10 sessions for speech-language pathology services

- 10 sessions for physical therapy, occupational therapy, and speech-language pathology services combined

- 2 weeks with authorization for continued treatment

- Care that adheres to the managed care organization's critical path (interdisciplinary treatment regimes that organize, sequence and time specific clinical interventions for defined patient groups)

4. **Managed Care Growth Trends.** A look at market trends helps us to appreciate the rapid growth of managed care. In 1996, HMOs covered 53.3 million Americans. From 1976 to 1995 HMO membership rose nearly tenfold. This trend is expected to continue well into the 21st century. It is predicted that HMOs will cover an additional 50 million Americans by the year 2000 (Spragins, 1996). Interstudy projections are that 103.2 million Americans will be enrolled in HMOs by the year 2000 (Interstudy, 1996).

   a. **Medicare managed care.** As of January, 1997, 5 million of Medicare's 38 million beneficiaries (approximately 13%) chose to join managed care plans (Shalala, U.S. Department of Health and Human Services, government employee correspondence, 1997). Medicare HMO enrollment increased by 54% from 1991 to 1994 (Kander, personal communication, 1996) and these patterns of growth are expected to continue concurrently with general managed care growth, as Medicare enrollment rates are highly correlated with total HMO market growth.

   b. **Medicaid managed care.** State Medicaid programs, which pay an estimated 50% of the nation's nursing home bills, are also moving toward managed care. This, too, is in response to rising Medicaid costs and state budget deficits. For example, Arizona uses a statewide contracting system to provide health care, including long-term care, through competitive managed care plans. The Arizona Health Care Cost Containment System (AHCCCS) is the first statewide prepaid Medicaid program. If Arizona is successful in moderating long-term care costs, other states can be expected to follow.

   A U.S. General Accounting Office (GAO) report on Medicaid in 1993 concluded that nearly all states are responding to rising enrollments and spiraling costs by establishing managed care programs (U.S. General Accounting Office, 1993). Consistent with the wide variations in Medicaid programs, Medicaid managed care is not a single health care delivery approach, but a continuum of models. At one end of the continuum are prepaid or capitated programs that pay a per capita amount each month for all covered services; at the other end are primary care case

Table 10–1. Some requirements of payers and accrediting agencies

Source	Requirements
Joint Commission on Accreditation of Health Care Organizations (JCAHO) (1997)	PE 1.3.1 All patients referred to rehabilitation services receive a functional assessment. TX 6.3 Rehabilitation restores, improves, or maintains the patient's optimal level of functioning, self-care, self-responsibility, independence, and quality of life.

The Rehabilitation Accreditation Commission (CARF) (1997)	6. A Medical Rehabilitation Program should demonstrate that the persons served are making measurable improvement toward accomplishment of their functional goals.
	
	33. The exit/discharge summary should delineate the person's:
	  a. Present functional status and potential.
	  b. Functional status related to targeted jobs, alternative occupations, or the competitive labor market.

ASHA Professional Services Board (PSB) (1992)	b. The plan for ongoing quality improvement periodically addresses all standards, with particular attention to services that are of high volume or that carry added risk, emphasizing Client evaluation and/or treatment outcomes; these may include, but are not limited to, identification of disorder, acceptance of recommendations, functional change in status, client/family satisfaction...

management programs (PCCM) that retain fee-for-service reimbursement with an added per capita management fee. Although prepaid models are still the most common, states are finding it easier to recruit providers to PCCM programs. As of 1993, two thirds of the states had PCCM programs. Medicaid managed care more than doubled between 1987 and 1992, and in 1993 included about 3.6 million recipients (or 12% of the Medicaid population). A 1995–1996 study of Medicaid managed care contracts by the Center for Health Policy Research at George Washington University found that nearly all states man-

Table 10–1. *(continued)*

Source	Requirements
Medicare Intermediary Manual (Guidelines) (1991) (See also Medicare outpatient billing forms 700 and 701)	Section 3905.3: Plan of treatment: The plan of treatment must contain the following: • Functional goals and estimated rehabilitation potential. . . , estimated duration of treatment A. Functional goals must be written by the SLP to reflect the level of communicative independence the patient is expected to achieve outside of the therapeutic environment. The functional goals reflect the final level the patient is expected to achieve, are realistic, and have a positive effect on the quality of the patient's everyday functions. Examples include: Communicate basic physical needs and emotional status (feelings). Communicate personal self-care needs. Engage in social communicative interactions with family and friends. Carry out communicative interactions in the community. 3905.4 Progress reports. Obtain: The initial functional communication level. The present functional level. The patient's expected rehabilitation potential Changes in the plan of treatment. [The medical reviewer may approve the claim if there is still a reasonable expectation that significant improvement in the patient's *overall functional ability* will occur]

date managed care programs for at least some portion of the Medicaid population (George Washington University, 1997).

B. Payer and Accrediting Agency Requirements

Although it is convenient to cite managed care as the impetus for change in health care, other economic and regulatory forces are also at work. As illustrated in Table 10–1, outcome-oriented standards are firmly established in accreditation agency standards and payer guidelines. They reflect a trend toward accountable care in terms relevant to a patient's everyday activities. Indeed, when one examines these standards and other requirements closely, they are not dissimilar to concepts of accountable and relevant clinical care beginning with documentation of baseline performance, establishment of a plan of care based on that performance, development of functional goals of treatment, reassessment of performance using the same baseline measures, and clinical decision making (e.g., continue treatment, modify treatment, end treatment) based on the findings.

In the requirements cited in Table 10–1, the emphasis is on "functional." The regulatory community operates largely with a definition of medical rehabilitation as "those services intended to optimize function." Thus, functional status measures have become the instrument of choice in documenting change. This is not, however, to be regarded to exclude other classes of measurement that are used for differing but equally important purposes. A functional measure can neither differentially diagnose nor identify patients' specific strengths and weaknesses. These needs must be met by standardized diagnostic instruments. Furthermore, functional measures may not capture all parameters of health-related quality of life, which are more adequately addressed by a growing number of psychosocial, wellness, and quality of life self-assessments. Many payers cannot appreciate the differences among these measures. Therefore, clinicians must inform payers of the various purposes of different types of assessment instruments, and explain that desirable outcomes can include more than functional skills.

III. CLINICAL CASE STUDIES

A. "Goodness of Fit" with Current Requirements

To examine whether five[1] of the case studies contained in this volume satisfy current health care requirements, I organized their key features by frequently reviewed standards of payers and accreditation agencies. This allowed an estimate of the cases' goodness of fit in a regulator-defined model of care. We might ask if these cases are reimbursable, and if they are not, what we have learned that can serve us in the future.

In Table 10–2, five case studies are summarized according to a core of current requirements by major payers and accreditation agencies. These requirements are:

---

[1] The other three case studies in this volume were not analyzed for their "reimbursable" features because they were conducted primarily for research purposes and were not intended to be used as examples of clinical care.

1. **An Expectation of Significant Practical Improvement.** According to Medicare, "significant" means a generally measurable and substantial increase in a patient's level of communication, independence, and competence compared to the level documented when treatment was initiated. Medicare does point out, however, that the term is not so stringently defined that it excludes a temporary setback or plateau in a patient's progress. A claim is approved if there is still a reasonable expectation that significant improvement in the patient's *overall functional ability* will occur. Overall functional ability defines the term, "practical."

2. **Establishment of Functional Goals.** Medicare defines functional goals as those that reflect the level of communicative independence the patient is expected to achieve outside the therapeutic environment. These goals are written to reflect the final level that a patient is expected to achieve. They must be realistic and have a positive effect on the quality of the patient's everyday functions (see examples of functional goals in Table 10–1). According to Medicare, functional goals may reflect small but meaningful changes that enable a patient to function more independently in a reasonable amount of time (e.g., the ability to indicate "yes" and "no," demonstrate competency in naming objects, use a basic vocabulary/short phrases).

   Because goals must be written in objective and measurable terms, documentation of functional goal attainment suggests the use of a growing number of reliable, valid and quantitative functional communication measures in the field. In adult aphasia, these tools include, for example, the *Communicative Abilities in Daily Living* (Holland, 1980; 2nd ed. in progress), *American Speech-Language-Hearing Association Functional Assessment of Communication Skills for Adults* (Frattali, Thompson, Holland, Wohl, & Ferketic, 1995), and *The Communicative Effectiveness Index* (Lomas et al., 1989).

3. **Estimated Duration/Frequency of Treatment.** This is the total estimated time over which services are to be rendered (i.e., duration), expressed in days, weeks, or months, along with frequency of treatment expressed in number of visits per week. The estimation is made at the outset of treatment and can sometimes be adjusted during the course of treatment if strong and justifiable reasons are explained in documentation.

4. **Patient/Family Input Into Treatment Plan.** National accreditation standards have been modified in recent years to prominently recog-

Table 10–2. Case study compliance with requirements

Case in Chapter #	Expectation of significant practical improvement	Functional goals	Estimated duration/ frequency of treatment	Patient/family input into treatment plan	Comparable pre-/ posttreatment measures to document change	Documentation of progress and relationship to functional goals	Patient follow up
1	+/– 1 month poststroke, young (37 yrs old), good health, severe, coexisting disorders	+ Obtain phonation Develop functional communication Reduce articulatory errors	+/– 2 mos/40 tx sessions	+/– Patient input No family input	PICA, WAB, Token Test, CADL, Apraxia of Speech Rating	+ Pt reported he was a better functional communicator Improved CADL score	+ 1 month post-tx PICA %ile retained
2	+/– 3.5 yrs poststroke, good understanding of problems, highly motivated, 67 yrs of age, significant improvement on WAB scores over 2-year period	+ Access semantic abilities through writing. Improve oral naming in conversation.	12 wks/11 tx sessions	+	+ Berndt Naming Task, structured naming (spoken and written) exercises (baseline, demo, practice, post baseline, conversation, homework)	+ Patient reported improvement, some changes in quality of life issues	+ Patient continued to be seen. 6 months posttreatment described, reports and demonstrates increased ability to retrieve words in conversation

	+/–	+	+	+	+	+	+
3	4 yrs poststroke, young (57 yrs), moderate aphasia, highly motivated, stimulable to treatment	Improve functional skills (e.g., driving golf cart, functional communication). Eliminate right neglect	7 wks/7 sessions	(Functional communication questionnaire)	Aphasia Diagnostic Profiles, battery of nonverbal tests	Eliminated right neglect (now able to drive golf cart) Increased ability to perform activities of daily living that depended on visuospatial and perceptual skills. ADP scores improved from 30th to 61st %ile	8 months after completion of treatment, ADP and cognitive test score gains were maintained
	+	+	+/–	+	+	+	+
4	6 wks poststroke, young (53 yrs), fair letter identification, absence of significant concomitant language or cognitive problem	Improve functional reading to allow return to work	6 mos/30 sessions		MTDDA, Boston Naming, RCBA, Grey Oral Reading Test, reading rate	Improvements on Boston Naming (from 52 to 55), Grey Oral Reading, and reading rate (from 12.5 wpm to 28 wpm)	1 yr posttreatment; working as independent plumbing contractor; made continual gains in reading with self-treatment

(continued)

Table 10–2. (continued)

Case in Chapter #	Expectation of significant practical improvement	Functional goals	Estimated duration/ frequency of treatment	Patient/family input into treatment plan	Comparable pre-/ posttreatment measures to document change	Documentation of progress and relationship to functional goals	Patient follow up
5	+/–	+	+/–	+	+	+	N/A
1.5 yrs poststroke, 63 yr old, supportive spouse, highly motivated.		Establish communicative connectedness as a couple Establish communicative ways of mutually resolving life's problems Establish chosen activities in life that further personal participation and independence	12 mos +		BASA, ASHA FACS, ABS, PWI, informal measure of interaction	Improvement on ASHA FACS (from overall score of 2.5 to 3.3) on Scales of Independence; ABS (from total score of 1 to 3), and informal measure of interaction	

Note: In Table 10–2, a plus (+) was assigned to each feature of the treatment that satisfied a given requirement; a minus (–) was assigned if the treatment feature did not satisfy the requirement. Because judgment often is exercised by accreditation agency site reviewers or health insurance claims reviewers in certain areas of decision making and because interpretations can be highly variable across health plans depending on their coverage terms and payment structures, a +/– was assigned to certain features with explanations offered. In one case, treatment was continuing; therefore, the requirement of follow up was not applicable (N/A).

nize the role that patients and their families play in ensuring that treatment is based on their individual needs. This is particularly true with the increasing cultural and ethnic diversity in our population. As clinical care embraces both medical and social science models, individual patient needs and preferences must be factored into each treatment plan. According to CARF standards, the family system is the focal point of services. Therefore, family members should be considered and involved as partners in all phases of a rehabilitation program. Often, patient and family input shapes functional goals of treatment (e.g., the ability to write letters to children in college or to dictate reports as a required job skill) and should be addressed in the planning phases of treatment.

5. **Comparable Pre-/Posttreatment Measures to Document Change.** Medicare guidelines clearly specify that speech-language pathologists may choose how to demonstrate progress. However, they emphasize that "the method chosen, as well as the measures used, should generally remain the same for the duration of treatment" (Section 3905, Medicare Intermediary Manual, p. 10–80). If the method used to document progress is changed, the reasons must be provided, including an explanation of how the new method relates to the previous method. The guidelines instruct claims reviewers to return claims if a speech-language pathologist reports a given subtest score for 1 month, then a score of a different subtest the next month, without demonstrating the two subtests' interrelationship. When this occurs, reviewers are unable to judge the patient's progress objectively. Use of comparable pre- and posttreatment measures (which can include alternate forms of tests if a learning effect could occur), therefore, will help to avoid the problem of returned or denied claims.

6. **Documentation of Progress and Relationship to Functional Goals.** Once again, Medicare guidelines state clearly that a provider must interpret reports of test scores or comparable measures and their relationship to functional goals in progress notes and reports. Simply reporting test scores without relating them to progress toward established functional goals may lead to returned or denied claims. Failure to specify this relationship leads to a "so what?" question, as reviewers are not able to determine the relevance of scores to desired functional gains.

7. **Patient Follow-up to Ascertain Long-term or Sustainable Benefit.** As the health care system begins to focus on more long-term cost savings, the issue of sustainable benefit becomes important.

Thus, the question of whether the functional gains are held over time is being addressed. As a result, a growing number of automated outcomes data bases involve data collection schedules that include patient follow-up (often 1-, 2- or 3-months postdischarge). The followup is conducted either by a patient visit with readministration of an outcome measure comparable to the pre- and posttreatment outcome measure(s), or by telephone interview of patient or family member. Payers are translating sustainable benefit data into the cost savings realized by lower utilization of skilled services because patients are less likely to need certain health care resources (e.g., home health care, family respite care, skilled nursing care, continued rehabilitation) if they remain independent.

B. Analysis

At first glance, the report card looks good. Most of the required features are present in these case studies. In fact, the clinical process illustrated by each provides a useful framework for clinicians who want to comply with current requirements as well as acquire data-based clinical knowledge. What remains questionable from a reimbursement standpoint, however, are the times postonset of stroke and the lengths of treatment. It is generally, although erroneously, accepted that maximal rehabilitation benefit occurs during the first 3 months postonset of stroke. Some may extend the period to 6 months. But we have learned here (and elsewhere in the professional literature in both group and single-subject experimental studies) that significant and functional improvements can occur long after the first 3 to 6 months poststroke, even with only a short period of treatment, as Case Studies #2, #3, and #5 illustrate.

This finding has important implications for the future of aphasia treatment, as well as the future of health policy development and negotiations with third-party payers. Its challenge, however, lies in discovering innovative ways to provide the treatment during a time when it is most effective and rendered in the most cost-effective manner. It is not simply *the length of treatment* but rather *the optimal timing of treatment* that defines good care by today's standards. Thus, the temporal aspects of treatment and good clinical decisions become indicators of quality care.

IV. A MANAGED CARE CASE EXAMPLE

A. What Might Have Been Done Differently?

Clinicians must develop effective strategies for working within a system of managed care. To accomplish this, they first must understand differences between managed care and traditional approaches to clinical care. The following case example, summarized from the ASHA publication, *Managing Managed Care* (1994), illustrates how services are being reduced:

The patient (FC) was a 78-year-old male who sustained a left hemisphere stroke with right hemiparesis and mild to moderate aphasia. Prior to the stroke, FC was independent and living at home. He was insured by an HMO that contracted with an individual practice association (IPA) to service Medicare patients for a capitated rate of payment for the full extent of health care.

FC was hospitalized for 6 days in an acute care hospital. During his hospital stay, he received SLP services, after which he was discharged home with home health care. Utilization review (UR) authorized a speech-language pathology evaluation, after which his speech-language pathologist was to send the report to UR for its review. Because UR had authorized only a single-visit evaluation, testing was abbreviated to what could be accomplished within the single session. FC had difficulty formulating both verbal and written language. Evaluation findings were as follows: FC's speech was fluent but characterized by literal paraphasias and neologisms. He could communicate basic needs at sentence level, but, longer, more complex utterances were difficult. Auditory comprehension was reduced to following 66% of three-step directions and understanding 50% of paragraph-level information. Reading was 80% accurate at sentence level, but FC was unable to read anything at paragraph level. Writing was severely impaired. He could write his name, but was unable to formulate written words or phrases. Before his stroke, FC had written letters to family members frequently.

On the SLP's recommendation, treatment was authorized, but for a limit of two sessions. Because basic needs were being communicated verbally and on FC's request, these sessions focused on writing skills. At the end of the two sessions, FC was able to write the alphabet and was beginning to write phrases when given a stimulus word. A home program was developed and his spouse was instructed to complete verbal and written exercises with FC.

On the basis of FC's progress and motivation, the SLP requested authorization for additional treatment. The physician who served as the gatekeeper requested copies of treatment notes and a progress report with justification for continued treatment, then forwarded the documentation to UR. Authorization was received for four more visits. At the end of the four visits, FC was formulating short sentences with 75% accuracy, writing the names of objects with 90% accuracy, and formulating and writing short sentences with 77% accuracy. His spouse was further instructed to use compensatory strategies and to encourage self-correction of errors.

Because FC was continually improving, the SLP requested four more sessions. Two visits were authorized with notification that no further SLP services would be approved. The last two sessions focused on family training. Further progress would depend on good follow-through by the family at home.

As a result of four separate UR authorizations, one evaluation session and eight treatment sessions constituted the posthospital SLP treatment program for this patient. This treatment program would be considered by many speech-language pathologists to fall far short of what was needed for this patient, particularly in the presence of continual gains. Another feature that interfered with a smooth course of treatment was the fragmented approach to authorization. In this example, the SLP was only given a few sessions per authorization in which to render service, never knowing whether treatment would be reauthorized. Consequently, a fragmented approach to treatment resulted. This might be an example of "living by systems." It is important to recognize, however, that in these times of change, systems are changeable.

B. Proposing a Different Course of Action

From the above example, some suggestions can be made for what might have been done differently to prevent an unacceptably brief and fragmented course of treatment:

1. **Understand the Practices of a Managed Care System.** Learn what drives decision making and who makes the decisions in a managed care plan. Once key decision makers are identified, effective negotiations can take place. Key decision makers include:

   • Provider relations managers;

   • Gatekeepers; and

   • Utilization, resource or case managers.

   The best time to negotiate a treatment package is before coverage terms are delineated or a contract is signed. Speech-language pathologists, working independently or collectively, can negotiate with decision makers at local HMOs or other managed care offices to reach consensus on service provisions.

   Provider relations managers are responsible for contracting with providers, and care management personnel manage the care of plan participants. Practitioners in hospitals could also discuss service policy with the hospital employee who is responsible for managed care negotiations, usually a vice president for managed care or the chief financial officer (Griffin & Fazen, 1993).

2. **Support treatment claims with data.** Once speech-language pathologists have the attention of decision makers, they need the support of objective data to support claims of acceptable levels of care. If 8 sessions are insufficient, SLPs must provide convincing data that demonstrate cost savings in other areas covered by the managed care plan or improvements in medical status, functional status, independence, and consumer satisfaction. Decision makers will respond to these areas, because these persons value economics and the areas translate into cost savings for the health plan.

A good resource for those seeking to work effectively with managed care entities is the Science and Research Department of the American Speech-Language-Hearing Association (ASHA), which has launched a major outcomes data collection effort under the auspices of the Task Force on Treatment Outcomes and Cost Effectiveness for use with managed care organizations and state/federal legislators. Several publications on treatment efficacy, cost/benefit, and patient satisfaction are currently available.

3. **Team with Physicians and Patients/Family Members to Advocate for Needs.** Clinicians can work with referring physicians and family members to ensure that an insurance company has an appropriate perception of a patient's needs. Such initial steps can avoid conflicts downstream, such as denials of treatment authorization requests as noted in the previous example. Consumers often are their own best advocates. Clinicians can inform them of appeals processes and of the right to pursue legal action, if options for rehabilitation are inappropriately restricted. Consumers can also get their employers involved. Large employers particularly have clout when they represent a large segment of enrollees in a specific plan. Consumer satisfaction is vital to financial viability for many plans, and they may adjust coverage to retain enrollees.

4. **Develop and Foster Acceptance of Critical Paths.** Another clinical tool that decision makers are beginning to accept is critical paths. If clinicians can provide a "map" that delineates the process of care with associated outcomes along a time line, which ideally is supported by clinical research findings, they may make considerable progress in adjusting overly restrictive terms of rehabilitative care.

5. **Educate Patients and Their Families About Managed Care Restrictions.** In a system of managed care, patient/family education becomes vital. From the outset of intervention, patients and families

should be advised of their plan's limitations and their options once benefits are exhausted. These options may include investigation of other sources of funding, self-pay, referral to a lower-cost clinic (e.g., university clinic), group treatment, or family or self-training to continue therapy. There should be no surprises that result in a premature end to the treatment program and leave patients unprepared to cope adequately with an impairment. Discharge should be anticipated from the outset.

6. **Explore Alternatives to Traditional Treatment Pratices.** Once options to extend treatment are exhausted up front, one must make the best use of what has been authorized by the managed care company. One questions if in the example, the chosen treatment approach was best given the circumstances. Other innovative methods that are of known or expected treatment effectiveness and efficiency might have been employed. These methods might have included a functional approach to treatment, training of family members as clinician volunteers, instruction of self-cuing, computer-assisted treatment, enrollment in a stroke club, or a homework regimen, in any combination that could be grouped into a brief treatment package.

It is admittedy difficult to change current practices given the intricacies of the health care service delivery and socio-political systems. The given suggestions, however, are meant as a guide directed toward extending the boundaries of traditional practice in the interest of consumer needs.

V. WHAT THE FUTURE HOLDS

Aggressive health care restructuring is expected to continue with major reforms, primarily in the form of prospective payment methodologies, slated for the delivery of medical rehabilitation (Table 10–3). Reimbursement restructuring for medical rehabilitation will extend across the continuum of care, from hospital, to nursing facility, to home health, to outpatient care. The new payment structures will continue to require change in the way clinicians render service. Outcome-oriented and streamlined interdisciplinary care are the expected by-products of restructuring. Delivery of service will move from discipline-specific care and toward an interdependent approach and multiskilling (a clinician or aide who is trained to provide a combination of services). Thus, research investigations, in addition to addressing general treatment effectiveness and efficiency, should address the role of multiskilled health practitioners and the effectiveness of their treatments as well as cotreatments provided simultaneously to a patient by different disciplines as lower cost alternatives to traditional care.

VI. RECOMMENDATIONS FOR CHANGE

The challenge for clinicians and clinical researchers is to provide care in the most appropriate setting; at the right time and intensity; coordinated with the best combination of professionals, support staff, and volunteers; at a low cost; and with the best outcomes. My recommendations for change address the current limitations of clinical practice and encourage the clinical community to discover new opportunities designed to either fit within or modify these limitations to foster care in the best interest of our patients:

1. Become knowledgeable about the changing health care system and its managed care structures and discuss the issues with key decision makers to influence change.

2. Develop and test new approaches to clinical intervention that embrace both social science and medical models of care. Beyond diagnostic and remedial aspects of clinical care, explore interventions that can occur outside the clinic and in a patient's community (e.g., address the need for adaptations in a patient's natural environments and interventions with a patient's family and friends or coworkers to enhance communication and, by extension, quality of life).

3. Apply what is known currently about treatment efficacy and effectiveness by reading peer-reviewed scientific journals, forming study clubs, and attending continuing education. Incorporate and test what is learned into current clinical practice.

4. Intensify clinical research efforts using both efficacy and outcomes research methodologies to document key outcomes (including functional communication and health-related quality of life) and disseminate research results in public forums, including professional journals, special interest newsletters, study clubs, and local, state, and national conferences.

5. Develop and test cost-effective alternatives to traditional practice including involvement of family members/partners in treatment, use of support personnel, and use of brief treatment packages, group treatments and cotreatments that have been shown to be efficacious.

6. Develop/use reliable and valid outcome measures in clinical practice and clinical research along the full continuum of the consequences of disease—from differential diagnosis and identification of specific strengths and weaknesses, to the effects of specific speech and language deficits on functional communication, to the

Table 10–3. Current and impending payment reforms for medical rehabilitation services

Payment System	Level of Care	Description
Diagnosis-related groups (DRGs)	in-patient hospital	A prospectively based reimbursement system, in place since 1983, that classifies hospital in-patients into groups, codified by principal diagnosis, and assigns a predetermined flat fee for the costs associated with hospitalization. The prospective payment system (PPS) has resulted in shorter lengths of hospital stay, delayed (or decreased) referrals to rehab practitioners, and a general reduction in utilization of services. As a result of PPS, the SLP's case mix in hospitals has changed notably, with dysphagia becoming the primary diagnosis treated. In some cases, SLPs report that 90% of the caseload in in-patient acute hospitals consists of patients with dysphagia.
Function-related groups (FRGs)	in-patient rehabilitation	A prospectively based reimbursement system that is being developed for in-patient rehabilitation, which classifies patients into function-related groups (on the basis of Functional Independence Measure [FIM] scores), and assigns a predetermined flat fee for the costs associated with in-patient rehab services.
Medicare salary equivalency	contracted services	In the fall of 1996, proposed regulations were written for the implementation of hourly reimbursement limits for Medicare contracted services. The earliest effective date for limits would be mid-1997. ASHA estimates that the SLP rate will be between $45 and $60, paid to a rehabilitation service contractor or individual contractor. Payment will apply to the time in a facility, not just treatment time. Supervisors will be paid a higher rate if on-site and engaged in supervisory activities at least 20% of the time. Large rehabilitation organizations that provide contractual services as well as private practices will feel the effects. They will be cutting expenses by reducing middle management and implementing other cost savings. Nursing facilities are already requesting adjustments of contractual payment rates.
Ambulatory patient groups (APGs)	out-patient services	For the last 8 years, Congress has been funding research for the design of a Medicare PPS for hospital out-patient services. Health Care Financing Administration (HCFA) has been dissatisfied with the progress of research to date, but is under pressure from Congress to establish a system soon. "Soon" may be 1–3 years from now.

		This is another prospectively based reimbursement system that assigns a patient to one or more ambulatory patient groups and is also based on measurements of functional status. "Speech-language treatment" is one of the 297 APGs used to describe patient services. The APG system will likely assign a specific payment for each patient group for a 2–4 week period (probably 2). At the end of the period, the patient is reevaluated to determine is he or she qualifies for a higher or lower payment for the next period (or qualifies for another period of treatment). Decisions will be made on the basis of scores on a functional measure.
Resource utilization groups (RUGs)	nursing facility care	For the last 9+ years, Congress has been funding research in the hopes of establishing a PPS in nursing homes for Medicare as well as Medicaid (since Medicaid pays 50% of the nation's nursing home bills). Here too, Congress is getting impatient. This PPS for nursing home residents who are classified into RUGs is expected to be implemented in 1998.
		The PPS allows annual payments to SNFs for SLP, audiology, PT, and OT based on a combination of:
		1. A facility's average monthly rehab payments from a previous 12–month period; and
		2. The national average Medicare SNF payment amount for rehab services, adjusted for number of discharges.
		When the monthly allotment of rehabilitation funds runs out or is nearing depletion, the SLP must present a convincing case to the facility administrator for seeking priority over PT or OT services.
Prospective payment system for home care	home health care	This research is far from completion. Currently, there is no reasonable estimate of when a PPS would be established for home health care. What is known, however, is that the prospectively determined fees for rehab will be based on scores from a functional status measure.

Note. Adapted from "Federal Legislation and Other Federal Activities: Impact on Rehabilitation Service Delivery," by M. Kander, 1996, *ASHA Special Interest Division 11 Newsletter, 6*(3), pp. 15–16. Copyright 1996 by ASHA. Adapted with permission.

effects of communication disabilities on overall wellness and quality of life.

7. Increase predictability of outcomes through large-scale clinical data collection and analysis that address the average length, intensity and timing of treatment, and associated costs and patient outcomes.

In view of the changing health care system, agreement between economics and efficacy requires the collection, analysis, and use of treatment and cost data using agreed-on and sound research methodologies, and reliable and valid measures.There is a great need for a data-driven approach to supply some answers to questions frequently asked by those who have the difficult job of allocating shrinking health care dollars to serve the entire population in need.

VII. REFERENCES

American Managed Care and Review Association (AMCRA) (now American Association of Health Plans). (1995). *Managed health care fact sheet.* Washington, DC: Author.

American Speech-Language-Hearing Association, Ad Hoc Committee on Managed Care. (1994). *Managing managed care: A practical guide for audiologists and speech-language pathologists.* Rockville, MD: Author.

American Speech-Language-Hearing Association, Council on Professional Standards. (1992, September). Standards for professional service programs in audiology and speech-language pathology. *Asha, 34,* 63–70.

CARF...The Rehabilitation Accreditation Commission. (1997). *Standards manual and interpretive guidelines for medical rehabilitation.* Tucson, AZ: Author.

Donabedian, A. (1980). *The definition of quality and approaches to its assessment.* Ann Arbor, MI: Health Administration Press.

Frattali, C., Thompson, C., Holland, A., Wohl, C. B., & Ferketic, F. (1995). *Functional Assessment of Communication Skills for Adults.* Rockville, MD: ASHA.

George Washington University, Center for Health Policy Research. (1997). *Negotiating the new health system: A national study of Medicaid managed care contracts.* Washington, DC: Author.

Griffin, K., & Fazen, M. (1993, winter). A managed care strategy for practitioners. *Quality Improvement Digest.* Rockville, MD: American Speech-Language-Hearing Association.

Health Care Financing Administration. (1991, June). Medicare intermediary manual, Part 3—Claims Process, section 3905, Medical review Part B, intermediary outpatient speech-language pathology bills. [Transmittal no. 1528]. Washington, DC: U.S. Government Printing Office.

Holland, A. (1980; in press). *Communicative Abilities in Daily Living.* Austin, TX: Pro-Ed.

Interstudy. (1996). Projections of HMO growth: 1996–2000. Chicago: Author.

Joint Commission on Accreditation of Healthcare Organizations. (1997). *Accreditation manual for hospitals.* Oakbrook Terrace, IL: Author.

Kander, M. (1996, November). Federal legislation and other federal activities: Impact on rehabilitation service delivery. *ASHA Special Interest Division 11 Newsletter, 6*(3), 15–16.

Lomas, J., Pickard, L., Bester, S., Elbard, J., Finlayson, A., & Zoghaib, C. (1989). The Communicative Effectiveness Index: Development and psychometric evaluation of a functional communication measure for adults. *Journal of Speech and Hearing Disorders, 54,* 113–124.

Spragins, E. (1996, June 24). Does your HMO stack up? Special Report. *Newsweek.* 56–63.

U.S. General Accounting Office. (1993). *Medicaid: States turn to managed care to improve access and control costs.* [GAO/T-HRD-93-10]. Washington, DC: Author.

INDEX